The Power and Simplicity of Self-Healing

My Journey from Life-Threatening Illness to Vibrant Health

Liberty Forrest

Contents

Introduction   v

Chapter 1   1
Chapter 2   10
Chapter 3   22
Chapter 4   31
Chapter 5   37
Chapter 6   44
Chapter 7   51
Chapter 8   61
Chapter 9   68
Chapter 10   73
Chapter 11   80
Chapter 12   90
Chapter 13   100
Chapter 14   106
Chapter 15   113
Chapter 16   123
Chapter 17   131
Chapter 18   139
Chapter 19   149
Chapter 20   155
Chapter 21   164
Chapter 22   171
Chapter 23   180
Chapter 24   188
Chapter 25   196
Chapter 26   201
Chapter 27   209
Chapter 28   216
Chapter 29   225
Chapter 30   230
Chapter 31   241

Bibliography   249
About the Author   251

Introduction

We've all heard those occasional stories of people who have recovered from untreatable or incurable conditions. There are those who were told they would never walk again — but through sheer determination, they did it. There are those who were riddled with malignant tumours and given a death sentence, but repeatedly visualised perfect healing and they became well.

There are numerous documented reports like these and usually, we think they are flukes, coincidence, or perhaps "miracles". They are so rare and so powerful, the notion that this could be commonplace does not occur to us.

But it should.

The "default setting" for any living organism is survival, yet it is only possible if the organism is inherently able to heal. We think nothing of our ability to recover from illnesses, injuries, broken bones. But why stop there? Why is it impossible to believe that we can heal ourselves of anything more serious than a broken arm or a really bad flu?

It is only because we have not known we could do it. For thousands of years, we have turned to medicine men, healers of all kinds throughout the ages, unaware that each of us possesses the power to create — and to heal — many of our illnesses.

The Power and Simplicity of Self-Healing is chock full of fascinating information that revolutionises the way we look at illness and healing. This life-changing book encompasses a wide range of seemingly disconnected and unrelated subjects, yet each one is a separate piece of an incredible and complex puzzle. I will explain each of them one at a time, ultimately revealing a startlingly simple picture that provides evidence that all of us have the ability to heal ourselves of more than we might think.

For most of my life, I suffered with ill health, some of it life-threatening, much of it just plain miserable and debilitating. For a number of years, I had found great help with homeopathy, believing it to be the be-all and end-all in healing. Although it is extremely powerful and produces miraculous cures, I reached a point where it was no longer helping, nor was anything else.

I had run out of hope and any reasonable options. My desperate and futile search for wellness took me down many paths from the conventional to the near insane. When it seemed all avenues had been exhausted, in an explosive moment of anger and frustration, I vowed to find a way to heal myself, believing that if other people have done it, then I could do it, too.

Along with sharing my personal story, this book covers a multitude of topics in a step-by-step systematic fashion, layering one piece of information on another and building a strong foundation so that all of the pieces are well-connected and logical.

Drawing on a wealth of information from numerous medical

professionals, researchers and scientists, along with the metaphysical, mysterious and inexplicable, I will drop one fascinating piece of the puzzle after another into its rightful place, creating multi-faceted evidence that self-healing of many of our ailments and illnesses is not only possible and powerful, but can be simple for anyone to do. If I can do it, maybe you can, too.

Chapter One

Everything changed that day. There was no big event. No fanfare. Nothing in particular that would precipitate such a monumental, yet invisible change. To everyone around me, everything looked the same. Everything *was* the same. But they didn't know what I knew. I was going to die. And soon.

For some years, my body had been doing its level best to leave this life. Until that day, my spirit had refused to allow it, a silent tug-of-war taking place deep inside me, my body winning one battle, while my spirit won the next. Back and forth, the war raged on. Just who would ultimately win was anyone's guess.

Until that day.

That day, I decided I would win. I would be victorious. It would be neither my body, nor my spirit that won the war, but my own determination that would stop it. No longer would I be the silent bystander, tormented by my physical pain and suffering, yet forced to continue to endure it by my ever-present and bloody-minded spirit that refused to let me die in peace. No longer would I tolerate the confusion, the not-knowing, the indecision and constant wondering which way this would turn out.

I wanted peace. I'd spent 40-odd years fighting for it but all I'd got for my efforts was more struggle, more suffering, and more pain. The only way to get that peace, the only way to end this raging war was to take matters into my own hands. I'd tried many conventional and alternative treatments for such a long time, all of which had failed. Finally, I'd found the answer.

It had come to me quietly, and ever so easily. One moment there had been unending suffering and misery; the next, there was the most powerful and empowering feeling of peace I'd ever known. Without effort, without decision, there it was: the startlingly simple solution.

I didn't think of it as suicide. I was simply going to end my suffering, for which there was no apparent cure. I believed I was doing everyone around me a huge favour, too, ending their suffering as much as my own because after several years, it had become quite a strain on my family to watch me deteriorate before their very eyes.

My children were constantly wondering which day they would come home from school and find me dead. My marriage was a mess, despite all my attempts to fix it, and I figured my husband would be better off without me. I was certain that everyone had had enough of seeing me lying in bed, unable to participate in even the simplest activities much of the time. I was missing the lives of everyone I loved. I was dead but still breathing. There didn't seem to be any point to my existence. I felt like a gangrenous limb in the lives of everyone I loved, creating an insidious toxicity of worry, fear, and resentment that was slowly poisoning their peace, their happiness, and their futures.

Thallium scans showed scarring and dead tissue from heart attack damage. But my heart wasn't functioning well and I'd had enough of the painful and debilitating symptoms of severe unstable angina. Between that and various other ailments, I hadn't lived a normal life for such a long time, I didn't even know what that meant anymore.

To make matters worse, for the better part of that year I had been suffering with trigeminal neuralgia, an excruciating, burning, gnawing pain that covers about half the face and head. It is said to be one of the most painful conditions known to humankind. I remember wanting to dig my long fingernails into the side of my face and tear it out. I understood how a trapped animals can gnaw off a leg. And I understood how people could literally be driven insane from pain.

It is no coincidence that this horrific pain on the side of my face was on the heart meridian, according to traditional Chinese medicine. My heart was struggling to get enough oxygen on a regular basis and the resulting pain and pressure in my chest and left neck were instantaneous. I had trouble breathing. Sometimes the pain spread to my left jaw and arm.

As a practicing homeopath, I kept vials of heart remedies with me at all times, as one dose would ease the symptoms as quickly as a sublingual blast of nitroglycerine, but thankfully, without its trademark explosive headache.

Within seconds of these all-too-familiar symptoms flaring up, the pain in my face would begin to scream. Or vice versa. It might be the facial pain first, followed almost immediately by a severe angina attack. Nothing I did made any difference. No painkillers, no remedies. I had the occasional brief reprieve, perhaps for minutes or even hours. But for the most part, I felt as though I had a burning hot poker jammed into the side of my face almost constantly, day and night, for nearly a year.

I'd had unstable angina for a few years before that. It was miserable but I had periods of improvement when remedies worked briefly and gave me a bit of hope that maybe the nightmare was over. I was able to function, keep my home and family running, getting through the bumpier periods and grateful for the better ones. And then the trigeminal neuralgia began, sending me into a whole other level of pain and suffering that was nothing short of pure torment.

* * *

I was surprised to discover how many people thought a diagnosis of angina was no big deal — myself included. It was just a "little heart problem". Firstly, I'd like to know how any heart problem is "little". Secondly, angina is a symptom of advanced heart disease. An attack of angina occurs when the heart is deprived of oxygen. This produces symptoms of pain and pressure in the chest and nearby areas and can become a heart attack. As with the rest of the body, if the oxygen deprivation goes on long enough, tissue dies. In the case of the heart muscle, eventually, it can no longer function properly and it stops.

Stable angina produces symptoms in certain situations or conditions, such as with exertion, emotional stress, or in extremes of hot or cold weather. Unstable angina produces symptoms without any provocation whatsoever. A patient may be feeling quite calm, perhaps lying down and relaxing, or even sleeping. Yet suddenly, blood flow is restricted and the heart struggles for oxygen. It can occur at any time, for no particular reason.

This is an extremely high-risk situation, as it can mean a heart attack is imminent.

That was how I'd been living almost constantly for a few years years. It was only because I was a homeopath and had a wealth of remedies available to stave off the worst of the symptoms that I managed to continue to breathe. But I hadn't yet found the remedy that would cure the problem.

The trick with homeopathy is that because it is a highly individualised and complicated science, it can be difficult to find the correct remedy. Each one has a central theme, at its heart a core mental or emotional issue or susceptibility that causes symptoms. The homeopath must take a very detailed history of the patient's life, as well as his complete mental, emotional and physical make-up, and then try to figure out the issue that lies at the heart of the case.

Only then can one of thousands of remedies — and its many potencies — be matched to the patient. Sometimes this is relatively straightforward but more often than not, as we are rather complicated beings, it can be quite a challenge. The more complex a person's life and symptoms, the more difficult it can be to wade through an enormous amount of detailed information and find the one piece that matters most.

Knowing that it is possible for homeopathy to cure all diseases, but not all patients, after so many failed remedies I was beginning to think I might be one of those unfortunate people for whom there was no hope. There had been so many problems and crises throughout my life, apparently it was impossible to see the forest for the trees. That one specific issue eluded not just me, but every other homeopath I had asked for help.

Aside from myself, there were only a couple of homeopaths in Calgary, where I lived, and although they had been able to help me with a long list of other ailments, the heart problem had proved itself to be even more stubborn than I was (which I hate to admit is saying something). I'd even sought the advice of some of my colleagues, people with whom I had studied, yet none of their suggestions worked either.

As the heart disease progressed and my health continued to worsen, I grew weaker not only physically, but emotionally and spiritually as well, until finally, I could not take it any longer. There was only one way my suffering was going to end, and the answer drifted silently and easily into my painful existence one blessed morning. I decided that I could put on my runners and go to Fish Creek, my favourite place to walk. It wouldn't take much to trigger another heart attack; a short little jog ought to do it. I could just wander off a short distance into the trees, just far enough to minimise the chance of anyone spotting me immediately and ringing an ambulance, but not so far that I wouldn't be seen before the coyotes got to me. My suffering would be over, and my family would be spared the knowledge that I'd been the one to end it.

In the meantime, I was still helping my patients. I was a dismal failure in my personal life, disappointing my family and causing them all sorts of stress. But in my professional life, several hundred people needed my help. As long as I was still useful, I could hang on a little longer. At least I had my plan. I knew that when I reached my absolute limit, I had a way out.

* * *

I must add — I've been reluctant to write about this because I don't want to give the impression that this is a viable solution of answer for ANY difficult situation. IT ISN'T. Suicide is NEVER a good idea. No matter how dark things seem, get help. Call someone. Speak up!

And my story is precisely why it's important to never give up. That's a big part of why I'm telling it. Read on...

* * *

Meanwhile, on my two or three workdays each week, I would put on some make-up in hopes of looking less ill. And because even then I didn't exactly look the picture of health, I always had an excuse for my patients. Late nights, early mornings, whatever. I would stumble down the hallway from my bedroom to my home office, get through an appointment, and fall back into bed until the next patient arrived.

But how bizarre those appointments were. I kept several vials of heart remedies on my desk and all too frequently, with a patient sitting across from me, I felt that familiar crushing pain in my chest.

I'd be listening attentively to a patient, asking all the right questions, taking notes — and wondering if this bout of angina was quietly becoming another heart attack. When my left jaw began aching, and pain radiating down my arm, I'd reach for a remedy, pop a little pellet under my tongue, and get back to my notes, all the while praying that I wouldn't drop dead in a patient's presence.

So despite my body's desperate efforts to die, I was still useful. That kept me going. The great relief that came with my plan on That

Day allowed me to hang on a little longer. At least I had a way out. And I would take it when I was ready.

A few weeks prior to That Day, I'd attended a week-long homeopathy workshop in Ontario, which was led by the principal of the school from which I received my training. A brilliant homeopath, he had taught many of the people who wrote our homeopathy textbooks. I knew that if anyone on the planet could find the correct remedy (which is an art as much as it is a science), it would be this man.

Because I was deathly ill and had run out of other options, he had kindly agreed to see if he could help me while he was in Canada. But as he lived in England, and at that time I did not, he said this would be a one-off session. There would be no second chance to get it right.

It was my last shred of hope and I clung to it with a desperation that tore at my soul. The remedy he prescribed helped for about two weeks. It was the longest reprieve I'd had in a few years. I thought maybe — just *maybe* — this would be the one. Maybe I could actually be well again. Maybe I could have my life back. I hoped — and prayed — for the best. But before long, the symptoms returned with a vengeance.

I was devastated. I'd been dealing with this life-threatening and debilitating issue for years. With my doctor and two cardiologists, I'd gone down the road of numerous tests, including invasive ones and their nasty side effects. I'd tried acupuncture, a philosophy in which I believe but it was too time-consuming and expensive for the level of care I needed. I investigated various other treatments unsuccessfully, eventually stumbling onto homeopathy, and finding great healing for many of my other problems, and it also helped my family with some of theirs.

On top of that, I believed in homeopathic philosophy, which is about not suppressing symptoms, but rather, it is about curing the reason for them, and it did so gently, safely and often quickly. It was the only thing that made sense. To my mind, there were no other options. Over time, I had seen it produce miraculous cures for many ailments that doctors could not help in myself, my family, my friends and in my patients. I knew its potential. I knew its power.

As far as I was concerned, at that workshop, I'd had treatment by the best homeopath anywhere. And that treatment had failed. The correct remedy refused to be found. It seemed clear that I one of those incurable patients and had no choice but to suffer until one day, I would finally die.

Shortly after the workshop in Ontario, I had to attend a homeopathy seminar in San Francisco. I missed most of it because I was lying in my hotel room, surrounded by countless vials of remedies that were known to be good for stopping even massive heart attacks in their tracks. As usual, with almost constant crushing pressure in my chest, it was difficult to breathe. The pain and tightness kept inching ever upward, along the left side of my neck, until my jaw began to ache, soon followed by the all-too-familiar tingling and heaviness in my left arm.

I popped remedy after remedy under my tongue, praying desperately for relief, yet it never came. The most I could manage to hold off the pain in my arm and jaw. But still, the unbearable pressure in my chest continued, making every breath an effort, leaving me further exhausted. It was as though my life had become one long, slow motion heart attack with only one outcome that was taking its bloody time.

I remember lying there, alone in my room, wondering if I should ring the desk and warn them that their cleaning staff might find me dead. Afraid that they would ring an ambulance and that I would be forced into medical treatment that I neither wanted nor could afford (having heard the horrors of American medical bills), I chose to say nothing and take my chances. A glimpse at the grey, haggard face and sunken eyes that stared back at me from the mirror across the room told me those chances were not very good.

I began to ponder the process and procedures in such a circumstance as dying in a hotel room far away from home and in another country. I wondered how they'd ship me back to Canada. I thought about countless television shows I'd seen, in which a body is discovered. I found myself wondering, with nothing but emotionless detachment, what would happen when someone discovered mine. I had grown so used to contemplating my death during years of living with a life-threatening ailment, often so ill I wondered if I'd last the next ten minutes, I was not at all frightened.

In fact, as I had done so many times before, I found myself wishing my heart would just bloody well stop and get it over with.

And then I cried. Not because I thought my heart would stop, but because I feared it wouldn't.

Chapter Two

It has been many years and several lifetimes since that horrible time. As if I hadn't been to hell and back on enough occasions prior to that, there were many more to come. Apparently, I wasn't through yet.

Obviously, I survived San Francisco. And a whole lot more, although it's nothing short of a miracle as I'd been so ill and for such a long time. I've travelled a rough road since then, in more ways than one, a road with numerous peaks and valleys, twists and turns. One day, I reached a point where right there in front of me, there was a sheer drop off a cliff, nowhere else to turn, nowhere to go for help.

I was angry. I mean, really, *really* angry. I was completely fed up with being sick and restricted by numerous limitations because of health problems. And that's when I began my journey of self-healing. I wasn't about to slip into those running shoes and go for a little jog in the woods anymore. I had too many reasons to live. Plus I was just too darned stubborn to give up.

All those years earlier, the Fish Creek plan had drifted ever so gently into my life just a few days after my return from San Francisco, bringing with it the sweetest relief I had known for some time.

Unbeknownst to any of my patients, they had kept me from carrying out my plan. They had saved my life, one agonising day at a time, until finally, I pulled myself out of that suicidal hole several weeks later.

I'd continued putting one foot in front of the other and waiting. For what, I didn't know. A cure? No. I'd given up on that ridiculous notion. That was obviously impossible. A miracle? Nah. I was pretty sure that wasn't gonna happen for me. I was getting on with my life and in the background, I was waiting. I suppose I was waiting to die.

A few months on, I endured a tormented night of hell like no other. It was far worse than anything I had experienced before it. I did not sleep. I wouldn't have believed my suffering could have got any worse than it had done over the previous year, but that night it reached a whole other level of unbearable. While my husband and children slept, I sat on the floor of my office the whole night through, alone and crying amidst stacks of homeopathy books. I was just about out of my mind, trying to read, trying to find an answer, and so desperate I didn't know what to do with myself.

To make matters worse, things were so terrible with my husband and his... let's just say, "extremely undesirable treatment of me"... we hadn't been speaking in recent days. It didn't help that he was already impatient with my health issues; I couldn't go to him that night even for a bit of comfort.

Fervently, I prayed to a God I thought either did not exist, or one who had abandoned me. I begged to *please* be shown what I had missed, what it was that I had still been unable to find after these years of suffering. Countless vials of remedies were strewn everywhere as I tried this one and that, a panic growing inside me like never before.

Eventually, too exhausted to even cry anymore, I collapsed on the floor, softly whimpering, utterly broken. I couldn't believe that I'd still not managed to find the remedy that would cure me. Perhaps I needed a remedy that had not yet been discovered, as was suggested by one of my homeopaths. Such a despairing thought! It had never occurred to me until he said it, and how I wished he hadn't.

As I lay on the floor just before dawn on that frosty winter morning, I considered giving up and going to hospital. I thought perhaps I ought to just let them do whatever terrible things they would do to me, angioplasty, bypass surgery, heart transplant — whatever. I had no more fight in me. I didn't care anymore. Nothing else was working. I'd lost all the battles, and all that was left for me to do was to forfeit and lose the whole damned war.

I was so ill, so emotional and terribly sleep-deprived, it was not safe for me to drive. And given that my husband and I weren't speaking at that time and I didn't feel safe to go to him with my troubles, I was not about to ask him for any assistance. I'd seen the results of that before, and I was in no shape to put up with it that day.

I considered ringing an ambulance.

I was utterly terrified. There was no part of me that wanted anything to do with conventional medicine. Yes, it has its place. Homeopathy, acupuncture or other alternatives are not going to help if you're in an accident and have a gaping wound or bones sticking out of your skin.

However, in so many other ways, I did not believe in its philosophies or practices. But on that terrible morning, I felt as though I had no other option. In fact, I believed that in the long term, it would do me more harm than good. In the short-term, though, it might give me some temporary relief before I would die. I tried to talk myself into making that call, but fear and a tremendous sense of dread stopped me. Always one to investigate Things Medical, I had too much information about the likely procedures and possibilities for surgery and other treatments to know they weren't for me.

I could not pick up that phone. Yet neither could I go on for even one more minute as I was. I had reached a critical turning point.

As I lay there, trying to muster the courage to ring for an ambulance, I considered just what it was that I found to be so frightening. I knew that when the ambulance arrived, the paramedics would give me something to thin my blood to prevent clotting. They would also give sublingual nitroglycerine to stop a heart attack, and morphine for the pain.

There was absolutely no chance that I would allow them to give me any of these drugs. I would only allow them to transport me to hospital. But perhaps they would not let me refuse. I didn't know if that was possible but I wasn't willing to risk it. Hmmm. Perhaps I would try to sleep for a while and drive myself to hospital later.

Lying on my office floor in the darkness of that early January morning, I did my best to prepare myself for what they would do to me once I was in hospital. It's kind of funny to think back on that now. I mean, if I was freaking out about a few drugs in an ambulance and knew I wouldn't allow those, what did I think would happen in hospital?

I'm chuckling on remembering that, but I guess the emotion, desperation, and sleep-deprivation must have messed up my ability to think clearly.

Anyway... as I'd already had extensive testing in previous years, including echocardiogram, ECGs, Holter monitor and thallium scans, I knew they would insist upon the next step, the one my cardiologist had been pushing me to take some time before — and I had repeatedly refused. They would order an angiogram, subjecting me to having a catheter shoved into an artery that leads to my heart, loading me up with drugs, and that horrible radioactive dye, which can cause kidney failure and heaven knows what else (oh, and death).

I panicked, there in the dark, just contemplating such violation of my body by tubes and toxic substances. It was not just a fear, not just distasteful. I was horrified at the very idea. I felt *violated* through to my soul just thinking about what they would do to me in hospital.

And that's when the light went on.

I had been praying to be shown what I had missed. Whether or not God was really up there, I had just been given an answer I had never found before. Maybe this was what I'd been missing.

Over the previous few years, I had wondered about a particular remedy several times, a sort of brief contemplation about it possibly being The One. But as none of my homeopaths or colleagues had ever suggested it, I had dismissed it without a serious look.

The centre of this remedy is about feeling violated. It does not have to be sexual violation, although I'd had plenty of that in my past, as an adult and going right the way back to my earliest childhood memories. I had taken other remedies that covered issues of abuse, but as with all remedies, each had a different central theme (for example, feeling inadequate, not wanting to be hurt, or feeling abandoned).

None of the others had worked to relieve my heart problem. Was this my magic bullet?

I knew this remedy had a strong affinity for nerve problems, which was consistent with the trigeminal neuralgia. Check. It doesn't have a backbone and bends over backward to please. That had always been a huge problem for me. Check. This remedy is terrified of injury, and of confrontation. Check, check. It has even got addiction issues, and I'd struggled with those in the past, too. Big check.

A new wave of hope raced through me as I scrambled to a seated position, grabbed my books and searched my repertory, which details even the tiniest and most bizarre symptoms, and lists all remedies known to cure each one.

It took some digging but I managed to find trigeminal neuralgia buried amongst the thousands upon thousands of "rubrics" (symptoms) in the repertory, and out of curiosity, I poked around and checked out 45 symptoms that I'd had either at that time or in the past. This particular remedy was found in 42 of them.

And so, on that frozen January morning, I took a dose of it in a fairly high potency, in keeping with the intensity of my symptoms.

As had happened with certain other remedies, the worst of my symptoms disappeared immediately. But within hours, something else had changed. I couldn't put my finger on it, yet there had been a significant shift in my energy. I knew this was a positive sign, although I was too afraid to hope I had actually found the cure. Perhaps it would just be another of those short-term reprieves.

Days passed, and then weeks. Soon it had been six months, eight months, a year, and I was still well. After years of torment, finally I had found the remedy that addressed and cured the reason for my symptoms. But for a long time, I was haunted by the memory of what I had endured. With the nightmare still fresh in my mind, I admit it was difficult not to wonder when it would return.

Gradually, the waiting subsided. Eventually, I didn't think about it at all, and I got on with my life.

I should have known it was too good to be true.

* * *

For five and a half years, I was completely well. And a lot changed in my personal life during those years. Along with the immediate disappearance of all traces of my heart troubles, it didn't take long before the remedy worked its magic on the mental and emotional issues that were behind my symptoms.

I mentioned about a key feature of the remedy being that lack of backbone?? Pretty shortly after taking it, I got one. Suddenly, I was being assertive. I stood up for myself, risked confrontation and eventually ended my unhealthy marriage.

I even ended up moving to England, a country that fed my soul and opened the most incredible doors for me. It was the first time I'd ever felt like I belonged anywhere — like I was home. Nestled into the English countryside, I lived in a quirky, beautiful, 500-year-old stone cottage called Ravenswood that was the most perfect dream home I could have ever imagined.

I was happier than I had ever been, or ever thought I could be. I tore around the UK and much of continental Europe quite regularly, going to France for dinner, Brugges for a day, Paris for an occasional weekend. With several countries so close and easily accessible, life had become one huge adventure. I was exploring not only the world around me, but my inner world as well. I learned all sorts of exciting and wonderful things about myself, and my abilities. I wrote three books in eight months. I began painting — and almost immediately, had my work in a couple of galleries and was having exhibitions.

As a lifelong psychic and medium, I'd always been aware of my evolving abilities but in England, I ended up doing reading professionally. I did "psychic phone-in" as a guest on the BBC every month or so for about five years. I took to the stage as a medium, connecting audience members with loved ones in spirit.

I was fearless during those years. And life was grand.

But then I received a couple of terrible and overwhelming emotional shocks. They shook me to my core, completely tore the rug out from under me, and smashed my life into a million tiny pieces. It was to be the beginning of yet another long period of extreme turbulence and distress.

Within a couple of weeks, quite suddenly and without the slightest warning, I had a massive attack of unstable angina. In minutes, the pain increased until it radiated from my chest to my jaw and down my left arm; I knew it was another heart attack. Years earlier, after finally settling into the belief that my heart was fine, I had stopped carrying remedies with me every time I left the house. Thankfully, when the problem returned so suddenly, I was at home. I took a remedy straight away and almost immediately, the worst of the symptoms began to subside.

In those terrible moments, I was launched back onto that desperate and frightening merry-go-round of ill health and a seriously ailing heart. I cannot find the words to tell you of the utter despair that swallowed my soul over the following weeks and months, when once again, neither my homeopath nor I could find a remedy to fix it for more than a brief period now and then.

Of course, I tried the remedy that had got rid of the problem the first time. No luck. It was no surprise, really. The reason for the previous troubles no longer existed. It wasn't about feeling violated —

which had been an issue since childhood and had continued right through to that previous marriage. The remedy had healed that issue.

This time, it was something else. And the specific center of my troubles was as clear as mud.

I resumed my desperate search for healing, but in the following years, grew even more disappointed and disillusioned than ever. I was so sick again and my heart was struggling to get enough oxygen. Just how it kept functioning was beyond me. Very poorly, obviously — and thank heaven for remedies once again staving off the worst of the symptoms. I found myself again just wishing for that time they would not work and that I could please, oh, please, just die. No, I don't mean I was suicidal — I wasn't — but I was deeply discouraged.

I felt worse in myself than ever before. I had got lucky once; I was certain I couldn't beat the odds a second time. My search for relief — for healing — was obviously an exercise in futility. And so, I prepared to die.

I went back to Calgary for what I believed was one last visit. I'd not been to visit my family and friends in a couple of years. Everyone could see how poorly I was. Over and over, I saw the looks of shock and concern. Those closest to me brought it up ever so gently; others merely looked as though they wanted to say something but didn't know what that might be.

I rested a good deal of the time, as I was too ill to do much visiting. I will never forget my goodbyes before boarding the plane to return to England. I was certain I would never see my children, grandchildren or beloved friends again.

Throughout my life, I'd heard or read occasional stories of miraculous and spontaneous healing against all odds. Many times, I became wistful and tearfully envious. What did those people have that I didn't have? Did they have special powers? Were they singled out by "God" or some other Divine Being who granted them healing because they were worthy? Were these incidents flukes, or were these people freaks of nature, who just happened to hit the healing jackpot for no apparent reason?

I'd endured so much — from the moment I came out of the chute, so to speak. I was tired — no, I was completely drained beyond all description. I just wanted peace. I wanted good health. The opportunity to feel well, do some good in the world, and simply enjoy this precious life I'd been given. Was that really so much to ask?

Apparently it was, because in my lifelong search for these, I'd been to hell and back several times, to no avail.

Somehow, in the couple of years after that terrible trip to Calgary, I limped along with my heart problem and numerous other long-standing ailments that added to the restrictions and difficulties of my life. I was used to living that way, but had grown very weary and found myself wishing I could just quietly slip away. I was not actively suicidal again; it was just that it was too hard to be here any more. I was sick and tired of being sick and tired.

On top of the ongoing turmoil and problems in my personal life, my poor health put me over the edge. I figured that if this was all I was ever going to get out of life, I'd just as soon be done with it. I didn't think I'd have to wait too long for that anyway, and that was fine with me.

Now and then, I continued to work with my dear friend and homeopath to find a solution, and tried various remedy ideas on my own. I found other new alternative methods of healing, too. As before, at times I had some improvements in one thing or another, but for the most part, I was still dealing with the heart problem, as well as restricting issues with painful and dislocating knees and hips, kidney weakness, loads of back and neck pain, sciatica and various other miserable conditions that I'd had for decades. I had been sleep-deprived for as long as I could remember, made worse by frequent and graphically violent and disturbing nightmares.

I was living with constant pain and exhaustion, even on my best days. I was fed up with having every aspect of my life affected by my physical health. But I knew I had a purpose in life, and I was determined to do my best to fulfill it. As tired as I was, I had to keep going. So I continued to try new and sometimes unusual methods of healing and doing my best to remain optimistic about having at least some improvement.

There came a terrible day when I had run out of reputable places to go, respectable professionals whom I could trust, and who might be able to help me. There was nowhere else to turn. I was stuck. With one dashed hope for recovery after another ultimately leading me nowhere and without hope, I slammed into a wall of desperation, of anger, and of complete and utter frustration.

After decades of suffering, I couldn't stand being sick any more. Hot, angry tears scorched my cheeks one cold winter day.

Suddenly, out of nowhere, rebellion bubbled up inside me like a volcano, erupting into something of an explosion of rage and frustration. Alone in my home, I spewed the words, "I'm fed up with this! I'm fed up with being sick! There's no one to fix it for me so I'm bloody well going to fix it myself! I have no idea how, but damn it, I'll figure it out!" It hadn't even been a decision; it was not a conscious choice. Quite simply, the words just fell out of my mouth.

And to be honest, there were some other, um, particular words that I don't dare repeat here. Oops.

As stubborn as I've been throughout much of my life (often to my own detriment), I can honestly say I don't believe I've ever felt such a level of determination as I did in that moment. I was furious. I'd had enough. I didn't care what it took, I was going to find the answers.

And find them, I did.

They did not come from one source. Nor did they come in one nice, neat package. Rather, countless puzzle pieces started appearing, as though pennies were being dropped for me to pick up. Individually, they were not particularly helpful. A new and interesting little tidbit here; another one there. Bits of information I'd known for years, some of which had been long forgotten — suddenly, they were popping into my mind and I didn't understand why. They seemed disconnected and entirely unrelated.

Until one day, a light went on. One day, there was that first "Aha!" moment, an awareness, the first link between two of the puzzle pieces. Soon there was another link here, and another one there, as random facts merged into little bubbles of information, most of which still had absolutely nothing to do with one another.

I had no idea what all of this would look like or what it meant. I didn't know what I was being shown, but it had become abundantly clear to me that I was being directed to these bits of information, and that it was going to be my job to connect the dots. I began keeping track of them.

In the weeks and months that followed, more puzzle pieces appeared out of nowhere, adding to the confusion by lengthening the list of unrelated bits of information, while occasionally, a flash of insight would bring several of them together, reminding me that I was, indeed, on the right track. There was science to back up speculation. There was documented evidence to support claims. There was proof; there was logic; there was reason.

Puzzle pieces began to fall into place. And gradually, everything settled into one fantastic, exceptionally powerful, but ever so simple concept: We have a far greater ability to heal ourselves than we might imagine. That includes me. And it includes you, too.

Excitedly, I began combining and using several of the elements of the puzzle, creating what was to be the earliest stages of my self-healing project, and taking notes of my progress. In a matter of days, I had achieved astonishing results, which, if I'm honest, I did not expect in the least. Certainly not to be as profound as they were, nor as quickly as they happened.

I continued to research the many "pennies" that were being dropped at my feet. I knew several people who were dealing with various ailments on all levels and decided to tell them what I was doing in hopes that they might want to be my guinea pigs. As the methods were so simple, they were all happy to say "yes". In every case, they noticed an improvement quickly, which continued as time went on.

The pennies kept dropping. I kept picking them up. And I carried on with my research. It became an incredible journey of learning and healing. The information and experience that I have accumulated could save — or at least improve — millions of lives by curing, preventing or even minimising the effects of many diseases. Whether you feel trapped by illness mentally, emotionally, and/or physically, there is a lot you can do to heal yourself. I understand if you're feeling a tad skeptical, but please bear with me. I promise I'll explain everything in great detail.

Sometimes, I look back and can hardly believe how ill I was. It went on for such a long time. It is astonishing that I survived but I reckon the Universe had a plan for me because it is truly a miracle that I am still here — and yet another one that I am as well as I am, even years later.

For decades before my angry declaration on that winter day, my journey to wellness took me down a twisted, winding road of treatments, from the conventional to the bizarre, while dragging me through the gamut of emotions. Fear, excitement, hope, frustration, exhilaration, disappointment, and wonderment — the road to healing has been fraught with steep mountain climbs, frightening hair-pin curves, plain straight stretches of no hope, no change.

Yes, there was an occasional reprieve, a welcome rest at the side of the road, none of which ever lasted. And I'd end up back on that path, searching, aching, certain — or perhaps just praying — that somewhere down that road, I would find healing. There had to be someone, something, somewhere...

Indeed, there was. I'd travelled such a long way, and for such a long time. And that road led straight back to myself. Just like Dorothy in the Wizard of Oz discovered that she'd always had the ability to go home, I discovered that I'd always had the ability to heal myself.

Perhaps *that* was the universe's plan. Perhaps *that* was the reason I survived — to be able to share tools that could help you heal yourself, too.

Chapter Three

By no means is my story of self-healing the only one out there. There are countless accounts of people bouncing back from terminal or potentially life-threatening illnesses, or accident victims who were told they would never walk again — and yet did. What makes my story different is that it's not just "my story, full stop." It's more than a timeline of going from critical illness to good health — without conventional medicine or doctors.

And no, I won't regale you with tales of a miracle healer appearing out of nowhere, waving a magic wand, and presto, I was fine. Nor will I claim I stumbled upon some Wonder Herb, diet, or religion that cures everything.

What I *will* share is far more useful — and far more logical. I'll take you through an intricate web of established practices and philosophies, studies, methodologies, healing modalities, and medical research. We'll cover a wide range of topics, from documented scientific evidence to the metaphysical and spiritual, and back again.

I highly recommend keeping a notebook handy as you read. There will be plenty of key points, tips, suggestions, and ideas you'll want to remember and explore. You might even find it useful to make a checklist of changes you want to try or topics to investigate further. In fact, this is more of a workbook than a "read-and-put-down" kind of book. I invite you to pause, reflect, and explore your own thoughts and feelings as you move through its pages.

If you have an "Aha!" moment, stop reading. Grab your notebook and write it down — in as much detail as you need. Don't trust that you'll remember it later. The book will be right here waiting when you return, and what you jot down may turn out to be important, as you'll see in later chapters. Be thorough, not hasty. There's no finish line to race toward.

After all, the point here is self-healing. It's a journey, a process. It takes time to dig in, to digest, to absorb new information — whether it comes from outside sources or from within your own thoughts and insights. You may find that by the time you reach the end, you want to start over again. The second time through, the pieces may fit together more clearly, and you'll absorb even more than the first time.

Within these pages, seemingly unrelated bits of information will connect, showing not just that we *can* heal ourselves from even the most serious conditions, but that we're designed to do so — and that, at its core, it's actually very simple.

So why is it so hard for us to believe? Especially when we already know the body has an incredible ability to heal? We've all seen "spontaneous healing" in action. Cuts, bruises, broken bones, surgical incisions — they heal. We endure flu, pneumonia, migraines, bronchitis, nosebleeds, stomach upsets — all eventually disappear.

We recover from surgeries and injuries, sometimes shocking ones, and marvel at the resilience of the human body. Yet we rarely stop to think *how* the healing actually happens. Why? Because it's what the body *does*. Such recoveries seem commonplace, not miraculous. We expect that after cutting open a brain or a heart, transplanting an organ, losing a limb, crushing a pelvis, sustaining a head injury with multiple internal traumas, or even undergoing a full sex change, the body will heal. We take it for granted.

Yet no one considers that neither science nor medicine can replicate what the body does. Doctors can repair, remove, transplant, stitch — but they do not make the body heal. That part happens on its own.

No one fully understands what knits our broken bones, or how cut skin regenerates. We accept it, because we've seen it work. Even when 75% of the liver is gone, the remaining 25% restores its function without regenerating — yet we accept that it works.

But tell someone they have cancer, MS, Parkinson's, diabetes, or lupus, and their first instinct is to turn to a doctor or some outside source. They believe they have no power over these ailments, that these diseases suddenly appeared out of nowhere to attack them. And in that mindset, the idea that they could *heal themselves* seems almost impossible.

And that, my friends, is a very big deal.

For as long as there have been doctors, or medicine men in various cultures, we've handed over nearly all our power when it comes to our most valuable asset — our health. Why? Because these "professionals" have spent years studying the physical workings of the body, and we assume they have all the answers. When they don't, we think it's because there aren't any. We believe them when they say there's no cure, or that we must follow a prescribed course of treatment, based on knowledge far beyond our own. We trust external sources, believing they know more than we do, believing that if healing exists, it comes from the outside.

Even worse, we often don't listen to our own bodies, with all their intelligence and innate wisdom. Our bodies know what they need, but when they try to tell us, we shove pills down our throats, push through exhaustion, ignore illness, and demand that they carry on despite long hours, poor diet, emotional stress, and a million other unreasonable expectations. And then we wonder why they start to break down.

When our cars break, we take them to mechanics. The mechanic diagnoses the problem and fixes it. We treat our bodies in the same way. Just as a musician is a specialist in music and an electrician is a specialist in electrics, we take our ailing selves to a physician, a specialist in the physical body.

But here's the thing: we are so much more than a bucket of parts. A broken-down car won't run if every part is fixed or replaced but there's no petrol in the tank. Even a brand-new vehicle sits silent until it gets that fuel. The mechanic doesn't need to look at the petrol; he just fixes the parts.

A physician does the same. He tests and examines the body, treating it like a mechanical problem. That bit isn't working? Give drugs, make it move, rest it, cut it out, or replace it — then the "vehicle" keeps going. He doesn't consider the energy source that powers the body, the life force that makes it move and function.

Physicians can recite long lists of ailments, injuries, and surgeries from which bodies heal on their own. They can explain the immune system, how white blood cells fight infection, how new cells grow to heal cuts, how bones knit and grow strong again, or how a single fertilized cell divides to become a fully formed human being.

But they cannot explain *how* it all happens. They focus on the physical and accept that the body simply does what it does. Full stop. Yet even though these processes happen everywhere, every day, they are far from commonplace. They are nothing short of miraculous.

If we don't think of healing as miraculous, it's because we've grown accustomed to it. Cuts mend, bones knit, colds fade, and we call it "nature." We may marvel briefly, then go back to our routines, leaving the body to do its magic — and, in the process, removing ourselves entirely from the healing equation.

To a large extent, we also remove ourselves from the illness equation. For minor ailments — colds, flu, small injuries — we usually attribute causes externally: a chill, a virus from a neighbor's kid, something we ate, being a bit run down. We trust that our bodies know how to heal and wait patiently, improving naturally day by day.

But when the diagnosis is serious — cancer, heart disease — we assume the cause is internal: genes, environmental toxins, or just bad luck. Illness becomes something that "happens to us." We see ourselves as innocent victims, under attack from viruses, bacteria, or tumors.

Sometimes people acknowledge contributing factors — a smoker linking cigarettes to bronchitis or lung cancer, or someone realizing poor diet and lack of exercise drain energy. But when someone like Miss Brown, the health-conscious tofu-eating neighbor, develops breast cancer, the shock is profound. We feel helpless, as if we are sitting ducks, waiting for our bodies to fail, powerless to intervene.

But here's the truth: we are *not* powerless. Not even close.

One of the fundamental principles of homeopathy — and indeed, many other medical systems, both alternative and conventional — is this: we have to be susceptible to an illness in order to get it. This applies to everything from colds and allergies to organ failure and depression. We are all born with certain vulnerabilities, which become evident as life exposes us to situations, substances, or triggers that reveal our susceptibilities.

Think of it like a dentist poking around in your mouth with that little metal tool, scraping and tapping each tooth to check its health. Most teeth respond nothing at all, but then — bam! — the dentist hits an infected root and suddenly you're flying out of the chair. The other teeth were fine; only the vulnerable one reacted.

Studies have shown this susceptibility in action. Researchers deposited the cold virus directly onto the nasal mucosa of volunteers — repeatedly. Only about 12% actually became ill. Chills, drafts, or other physical factors didn't change the outcome.

How can catching an illness not depend entirely on physical circumstances? Because the cause of illness is only *partially* physical, at best.

A bigger challenge in Western cultures — and perhaps one of the largest obstacles to healing — is the belief that the mind and body are separate. Conventional medicine further complicates this by treating the body as a collection of isolated parts: musculoskeletal system, nervous system, immune system, heart, lungs, kidneys, brain, reproductive organs, feet... the list goes on. We have cardiologists, podiatrists, ob-gyns, neurologists, psychologists, ophthalmologists, dermatologists, endocrinologists — each a specialist in their own corner of the body.

But we are not separate parts. None of these systems could survive on its own. Together, they make a whole person.

This may explain phenomena like phantom limb pain, where amputees feel sensations — itching, tingling, pressure — in a limb that no longer exists. Even missing organs can elicit "phantom" sensations. The reason? Each of us is a single, integrated being. Every part communicates with every other part. True healing requires addressing the whole person, not just an isolated symptom.

Hippocrates (460–377 BC), the Father of Western Medicine, understood this. He believed that the mind and body must be considered as a whole, and that the first principle of medicine is to respect and support the healing force inherent in every living organism — the force that animates all of nature. He taught that nature is the only true physician, and a doctor's role is to support the body's own natural healing power when it becomes weakened.

Hippocrates saw a physician's task as discovering the root causes of illness and health, taking into account all aspects of a patient's life, lifestyle, and environment. How ironic — and a bit tragic — that the man whose name still graces the Hippocratic Oath should have had such a holistic vision, while many of his modern-day counterparts do not.

Holism means that the significance of each part can only be understood in terms of its contribution to the whole. This is especially true in healing. We rarely get sick in just one isolated part. A patient may present with pancreatic cancer, an anxiety disorder, or psoriasis, but the truth is that the *whole person* is affected. The body communicates internally: cancer cells "talk" to liver cells, liver cells "talk" to blood cells, blood cells "talk" to brain cells.

Chemical messengers — neurotransmitters and neuropeptides —

carry messages of illness to every cell in the body, which responds according to its receptors. Research in psychoneuroimmunology explores exactly this: how the central nervous system, the neuroendocrine system, and the immune system all interconnect.

Even the CNS — one of the most complex systems in the body — begins with something as simple as a thought. Your brain is an enormous electromagnetic field, and thoughts produce electromagnetic waves. Astonishingly, these waves create chemical messengers seemingly out of nothing, which are instantly sent throughout the body and received by receptors on cell walls. It's as if thinking about baking a cake conjures the ingredients from thin air — except in this case, your thoughts are sending molecules that affect every cell in your body.

Previously, it was thought that the CNS operated as a one-way system, with neurotransmitters and neuropeptides staying confined to the brain. But that only tells half the story. Through multiple pathways — the bloodstream, the immune system, and more — chemical messages are constantly relayed from brain cells to receptors on cell walls throughout the body, and back again. Cells communicate with each other as well, because the body is a single, integrated unit designed to function as one.

Scientists have discovered roughly 60 different neuropeptides in the brain, and these tiny chemical messengers allow cells to communicate in four ways: brain-to-brain, brain-to-body, body-to-body, and body-to-brain. The messages they carry change constantly, fluctuating with your thoughts and emotions throughout each day, and these messages ultimately influence whether you become ill—or well.

Every thought, idea, or belief triggers an emotion, whether positive or negative, helpful or harmful, and each emotion carries a chemical consequence. Instantly, these chemical messages are sent to receptors on every single cell in the body. Candice Pert, a neuropharmacologist who has conducted extensive research in this area and authored *Molecules of Emotion* (as well as numerous scientific articles), proves that an inextricable link exists between our emotions and the regulatory endocrine and immune systems, mediated through the central nervous system. Her work confirms why expressing ourselves in healthy ways, and releasing negative energy before it builds up, is so important for our physical wellbeing.

It's easier to understand if we look at the fight-or-flight response. Strong emotions, like fear or anger, send powerful messages throughout the body, creating chemical changes in an instant. We are flooded with norepinephrine, a catecholamine that prepares the body for running away or defending itself.

Imagine a woman walking alone down a deserted street at night. She hears footsteps behind her, seemingly matching her pace. Glancing over her shoulder, she sees a shadowy figure just a stone's throw behind. Certain she is being followed, she perceives a threat to her safety. In her mind, she thinks: *"That man is going to hurt me."*

Instantly, adrenaline floods her system. Her muscles tense for action, her lungs draw in extra oxygen, her heart beats faster to circulate it. Through the mind-body connection, her fear has created chemical messengers that trigger a response in every cell of her body. Her fear is not just a thought; it is a full-body experience.

When the threat passes — the man turns a corner and disappears — her thoughts shift to safety. New chemical messages are sent throughout her body, and she can relax.

We often think of this process as automatic, and in many ways it is. But hidden within it is something extraordinary — a seed of power, the power that every one of us has to heal ourselves.

No doubt what I'm about to say will raise eyebrows, and perhaps even provoke indignation, but please bear with me, because this book will prove the veracity of my words.

Whether illness arises from an external source, like a virus, or an internal one, like cancer, sometimes it's because we have created the conditions in our bodies that allowed the illness to take hold. You may have heard this before, and you may accept it—or not. Either way, please just hear me out. I didn't like it the first time I heard it either, but it is just as true as the words you're reading.

I know what you're thinking (as I did when I first heard it): *How dare she suggest that I created cancer, ALS, suicidal depression, kidney failure, or anything else that might be ailing me?* Do I really think you want your illness? Do I really believe you wouldn't prefer to be well?

Hang on a minute. I have only said that we create every illness we get. I am not saying it consciously or willingly, nor that you woke up one morning thinking: *"Hey, today I think I'll develop a critical illness!"* I am not saying you enjoy being sick, in pain, miserable, or exhausted. If you did, you wouldn't be reading this book. It is true that some people do unconsciously maintain illness or even need to be ill for various reasons, but that is a whole other discussion — and another book entirely.

Here's the empowering flip side: if we can create illness, then we also have the capacity to create wellness.

And therein lies the most astonishing, life-changing nugget of truth: the very same mind-body connection that allowed the disease to appear is the one we can harness to restore our health.

So, now that you know the power is already inside you, the question becomes... what will you do with it?

Chapter Four

I'm about to take you on an incredible and fascinating adventure, one that adds layer upon layer of information until a beautiful portrait of self-healing emerges.

Think of it like standing nose-to-canvas in front of a painting. Up close, all you can see are individual brushstrokes — little dabs and blotches of colour that don't look like much on their own. But when you step back, the pieces blend and soften into one stunning portrait.

This book works the same way. Step by step, we'll journey through what at first might look like separate, unrelated pieces of a puzzle. Then, just as it happened for me, the light will go on for you too — and you'll begin to see how all those brushstrokes connect to reveal the power and simplicity of self-healing.

And like every great story, this remarkable journey has a humble beginning: a quick look at some basics about the human body. It's a miraculous thing, yet most of us rarely pause to appreciate it. I've thought about this a lot over my life — and I've made it my business to learn a fair bit about how it works. After spending so many years so ill, I developed a deep respect for good health and for the intricate brilliance of the body itself.

Of course, I knew the basics: without a reasonably healthful diet, some exercise, and adequate rest, we're all more prone to illness. Yet despite being mindful of those factors most of my life, I managed to be extremely ill anyway. Still, I always figured I would have been in far worse shape if I hadn't at least done what I could to look after myself.

But somewhere along the way, after decades of exploring "energetic medicine" like acupuncture, reiki, and homeopathy, and living as a deeply spiritual woman, I forgot about the importance of the physical. My whole world revolved around energy and spiritual matters.

I was a psychic and a medium. I'd discovered a natural ability as a "spiritual healer" — a conduit for universal healing energy, for lack of a better description — and I developed it (something you'll read about in a later chapter). I've always been sensitive to the "energy" around me, and I've lived by Pierre Teilhard de Chardin's famous assertion that "we are not human beings having a spiritual experience; we are spiritual beings having a human experience." My books, my art, my conversations, my very perspective on life were all built on a spiritual foundation.

The more ill I became, the more convinced I was that the answer to healing lay in spiritual or "energy" work — and the less I considered the physical.

Until I hit a crisis. Suddenly, there was nowhere left to turn and no one left to help me. I realised I was on my own.

I don't think I'd ever felt so alone. I was trapped inside this ailing body, doing anything and everything I could for so many years, yet still hurting every day. Still restricted by pain. Still unable to do so many of the things I longed to do. And there was no one to ask for help.

That was the point when anger rose up in me. I decided, enough. I was going to fix it myself. But where on earth would I even begin?

As I've already told you, homeopathy had made the most significant difference to my health, completely curing or easing many of my ailments. But constitutionally, I was not strong from the start. My gene pool wasn't great on either side, and my prenatal beginnings didn't help.

My mother was only 15 when she became pregnant with me. Still growing herself, she tried to hide her pregnancy by eating very little and received little — if any — prenatal care once her secret was discovered. To top it off, she smoked throughout the pregnancy, back in the days before anyone realised how harmful that was to an unborn baby.

All of this put me at a disadvantage from the outset. With the right care, attention, and a nurturing, positive environment, I'm sure I'd have been in far better shape than I was. But the emotional impact of a very turbulent life, first as a child and then as an adult, left deep, long-term scars.

After spending some time with my birth mother, I was taken from her and placed in foster care, until I was eventually adopted into an often angry and frightening environment. The emotional threats — along with physical and sexual assaults — did a lot of damage and left wounds far deeper than anyone could see.

As the years passed, I fought my way through one nightmare after another, living in a constant state of anxiety, always terrified for my safety and wellbeing. Somehow, I managed to emerge with great inner strength. Physically, though, I was a wreck.

Too many pregnancies for my already frail constitution — followed by life-threatening haemorrhages after two deliveries — left me with severely weakened kidneys. For decades, I spent far too much time running to the loo. Even short walks, errands, or shopping trips became awkward. At night, I was up every hour or two, my sleep constantly interrupted.

Then there were the car accidents. I'd been in a couple of major ones, neither of which was my fault, but my body paid a high price anyway. Years of back pain, neck pain, and violent headaches followed.

For 18 years I battled M.E. (or Chronic Fatigue Syndrome,

depending on where you live). I had migraines more days in a month than not, hormonal issues, endometriosis, and liver problems. I didn't know what it was to sleep well — or much at all. I was constantly exhausted, running on fumes.

Layer onto that depression, overwhelming anxiety disorders (more on those later), and a nine-year battle with anorexia. All of it wreaked havoc on my body, though at the time I didn't fully realise the extent of the damage.

Fast-forward to the point where I finally decided to take control of my health. That decision is what ultimately led to the writing of this book. By then, many of my ailments had been cured, but a stubborn list of nagging problems still severely restricted my life.

The most worrying issue — in terms of longevity — was my heart. The others "just" made every day a miserable challenge. On a daily basis, I lived with pain and extreme stiffness in many joints, as well as my neck and back. My right hip and knee dislocated easily.

For over 30 years, simply stepping out of my vehicle, walking down my own stairs, or getting up from a chair could trigger a painful dislocation that would take days — sometimes weeks — to resolve. I spent long stretches relying on crutches or a cane, both awkward and restrictive.

Add to this the constant hip and back pain that woke me several times each night, combined with multiple trips to the loo thanks to those weakened kidneys. I had been unbearably sleep-deprived for about 35 years — a likely cause of the relentless headaches I endured almost every day.

I dragged myself through life never knowing what it felt like to be rested, refreshed, energised, or even remotely well. I looked drawn and exhausted all the time. I stood up from chairs slowly and painfully, like a frail little old lady twice my age. People often asked if I was all right or if I needed help.

Meanwhile, at middle age, other people were out jogging, lifting weights, cycling, playing hockey. And there I was — unable to get out of a chair without appearing in distress. I had very little physical strength and no real concept of what "stamina" even meant.

But underneath it all, something stronger than my body remained. I had work to do. A destiny to fulfil. A life to live. And I had bloody well had enough of the limitations and restrictions imposed upon my damaged body for three and a half decades.

I remembered a meditation I'd done some years earlier — one in which I'd actually had a conversation with my heart. It was an intriguing experience, to say the least. One of the key messages I received that day concerned very specific emotional issues in my life.

As a homeopath, I already understood that physical symptoms can be a manifestation of mental and emotional issues. But that meditation spelled out some of the particular reasons for my heart trouble.

Some time ago, I came across the notes I'd made that day. It was clear that fear and denial had kept me from addressing those issues. It wouldn't be the first time, but I prayed it would be the last.

For most of my adult life, I had focused on health and wellness, determined to get it right. I crammed tofu, seaweed, grains, and piles of fresh fruits and vegetables down my family's throats. My children grew up believing that if they ate all their dinner, carrot sticks or fruit for dessert was a treat. There was plenty of time for them to discover cakes and other sweets later.

We didn't do fast food, junk food, or fizzy drinks. I got plenty of exercise, hadn't smoked since my teens, and rarely drank alcohol. I lived as healthy a lifestyle as I could manage — yet I remained ill.

I felt betrayed by my body. I was impatient, angry, and frustrated when it caused me pain, restricted my life, or when my heart symptoms flared up. It's ironic, really. I was so focused on making my body well, yet most of the time I was angry with it. I told it so, too — in no uncertain terms.

I pushed on when it hurt, believing that if I "gave in" every time I felt miserable, I'd spend my life in bed. I ignored what my body was trying to tell me and then was furious when it fought back.

It occurred to me that, on some level, I had disconnected from my physical body as a small child — perhaps an effort to escape my physical environment, the assaults and violations.

That day, as I sat trying to figure out how to heal myself, I realised all my various aches and pains were my body's attempts to communicate with me. Of course, I understood that the nature of an ailment is directly related to one's mental and emotional state. Pain that feels like pressure often reflects feeling pressured at work or at home.

But this was different. It wasn't just that my body was manifesting or reflecting my mental and emotional issues. It was trying to communicate with me.

For much of my adult life, I'd been a single parent with a job to do and a group of children counting on me. Through sheer determination, I had spent years ignoring my body and pushing through my physical pain. In some ways, that made me stronger mentally, emotionally, and spiritually.

But now I could see the other side of it. That same approach had allowed me to survive some very dark and terrible times — but disconnecting from my physical self had also created problems. Just how big those problems were, and how much damage I'd actually done to myself, I didn't yet know.

But having set out on this path of self-healing, I was about to find out.

Chapter Five

I am certainly not the first person to understand that our symptoms are our bodies' way of communicating with us. Many alternative healing practices, such as BodyTalk or Emotional Freedom Technique, validate this idea, and people like Louise Hay have been teaching it for years.

Even a doctor will tell you that pain is the body's way of saying something is wrong. It's not a new idea, but on the day I swore I would heal myself, it took on a whole new meaning. It was time to stop ignoring my physical body, to reconnect with it, to remember that it was just as important as my mental, emotional, and spiritual aspects. Without it, the others simply could not exist. It was time to stop being angry at it and start listening.

You might think it was my heart problem that pushed me to this point of determination, but you'd be wrong. Sure, it was still there, reminding me of its presence with unstable angina, keeping me at risk for another heart attack. But I wasn't as critically ill as I had been in the past. I was relatively functional — far from symptom-free, but able to manage.

My heart grumbled almost daily for no apparent reason. Angina flared with even minor exertion or emotional stress. Yet I had grown used to it and didn't expect it to improve. I figured my heart would gradually worsen over time and suspected I might only have a few years left.

Living alone, I was just happy if I could care for myself day-to-day. I knew my limits and made sure to respect them.

No, it wasn't my heart that led me down the path of self-healing and writing this book. It was something far simpler.

At that time, I was in the midst of a massive life overhaul. I had endured significant emotional trauma and loss, much of it because I had no choice but to leave England and return to Calgary. I'd never liked it there, and the idea of going back after living my dream life Across the Pond was dreadful.

But the economic situation in Europe demanded it. I ended up back in Calgary, having lost virtually everything I'd worked my entire adult life to acquire — my home, a thriving homeopathy practice, my vehicle, a house full of furnishings. There I sat in a rented flat with no job, poor health, no financial security, and no pension.

To make matters even worse, the emotional ties I had to England — and to so many people there — were incredibly strong. I had intended to live the rest of my life there and had even become a British citizen several years earlier. I had worked hard to plant roots in that country, and they were deep. Leaving was one of the hardest and most painful things I've ever had to do.

Seeing my family and friends in Calgary again brought some joy, but only in small doses. They were busy with their own lives, and for the most part, I was alone, stuck in a city I had always hated, living a ground-floor rented flat with a view of a car park, and where people could peer into my sitting room as they walked by, a mere ten feet away.

How I longed for Ravenswood, my beloved quaint cottage and English country garden! I kept the blinds closed almost all the time to preserve what little privacy I could, but it did nothing for my depression or my ability to heal any part of myself, or my life. Days would pass without me leaving my little box. I shut the world out as best I could, trying to cope with overwhelming homesickness on top of my physical ailments, all while figuring out how to start over.

One thing was certain: this painful move and heart-wrenching homesickness would not be for nothing. I was determined to put myself — and my life — back together in a stronger, healthier, better way.

At least I had begun meditating again, particularly practicing mindfulness meditation, which has been shown to offer a host of health benefits. According to Carolyn Schatz on Harvard Medical School's health blog, mindfulness meditation can help "...with so many physical and psychological problems — like high blood pressure, chronic pain, psoriasis, sleep trouble, anxiety, and depression. It's also been shown to boost immune function and stop binge eating."

Mindfulness teaches us to focus on this moment — right here, right now. Not a moment ago, not a moment in the future. A mind trained this way is a mind that does not allow anxiety or fear to take over.

The purpose of learning mindfulness during meditation is to work toward living mindfully in every moment of life. It's a challenge, yes, but a worthwhile one. Dwelling on the past or worrying about the future are habits that ruin the present and increase stress, which in turn worsens health.

Studies on meditation in general have shown measurable benefits: lower heart rates (reducing the workload on the heart), decreases in harmful stress-related chemicals, and a reduction in free radicals — those silent killers our bodies generate continuously (we'll dive more into them in later chapters).

It has also been proven to lower cholesterol levels and, in general, seems to slow the aging process. Not only do people who meditate regularly tend to live longer than those who do not, but they also report increased feelings of happiness and emotional stability, a stronger sense of self-worth and vitality, and improvements in memory and learning.

Once I was settled in terms of organising my flat and the business end of creating a new life after an international move, I resumed meditating first thing every morning, last thing before bed, and most days there was a candlelit mid-afternoon bath with soft music, during which I meditated on anything that I thought might help me feel better. As one of the best stress-reducers and coping mechanisms I have ever found, reincorporating meditation into my daily life went a long way to keeping me focused and functional when it would have been so easy to come apart.

Regular meditation was an excellent place to begin my self-healing project, but I knew my body needed some activity, too. That was the tricky part. Apart from some gentle Tai Chi off and on, for years I'd been spending my days reading and writing, working on my websites, recording meditation CDs, generally just living a sedentary life indoors.

In part, this was due to the troubles with my heart, but it was also because my hip and knee could dislocate so easily—a condition that was not serious but terribly painful. Many times I would set out on a bit of a walk to see what happened. Would my body be kind? Or would it betray me once again? More often than not, it wasn't long before that familiar old pain crept into my chest, or my hip or knee, and I'd have to turn back, disappointed, restricted, and trapped yet again.

Down the years, I stayed inside for longer and longer periods of time, as one of these ailments was always waiting to prove to me that that's where I belonged. I resigned myself to the fact that I was no longer able to enjoy going for walks, which I'd always loved, but even a leisurely stroll had become impossible most of the time.

I worried about my inability to get some exercise. I understood that this was not good for my mental or emotional health either. As I was reconnecting with my physical body after what seemed a lifetime of separation, I decided to take it for a little walk. Buoyed by my positive attitude and renewed determination to be well, come hell or high water, I went to Carburn Park, a favourite "nature spot" nearby.

It was a lovely winter day, sunny and crisp, not too cold. The pond was frozen over, but a little further on, the Bow River trickled along, clear, blue, and sparkling. There were some Canada Geese sitting on its snowy banks, watching the water meander around occasional slabs of ice. As this was an extremely emotionally challenging time for me, it did my heart and soul a lot of good to get out of my flat and be with water and trees for a while. Determined to lift my spirits and just enjoy the experience, and always one to throw myself in at the deep end and do everything "whole hog," I set out at a fairly brisk pace.

But it didn't last long. About ten minutes into my walk, there it was—the beginning of that old familiar pain in my right hip as it tried to dislocate itself. I knew it would only get worse, so I turned around immediately, each step more painful than the last.

I fought back tears of frustration as I went the short distance back to my flat, angrily wondering, '*How the hell am I ever going to be well again??*' I wanted to be well. I'd fought long and hard for good health for years. I'd tried so many different healing methods, had carried on working hard in whatever ways I could manage, and had used my determination to get me this far. Why couldn't I be well??

Someone suggested that I take herbs to try to fix the problems in my joints, but I rejected the idea based on my previous experience and knowledge. Although they have helped countless people, they had never done much good for me, and they were too harsh for my very sensitive body, too.

They are like drugs—not without numerous side effects and potential risks—and they can, in fact, be quite dangerous. The common misconception about herbs is that just because they are "natural," they are completely safe. This is a deadly myth. Take the rhubarb plant, for example. The roots are used for medicine. The stalk is eaten like a fruit. And the leaves will kill you. Medicine, food, and poison, all in the same plant.

St. John's Wort, an herb that many people have been gulping like mad for depression over the past couple of decades, can cause dangerously high blood pressure in some people when mixed with certain foods and drugs. One should never take narcotics, tryptophan, nasal decongestants, asthma inhalants, cold or hay fever medications, or diet pills whilst taking St. John's Wort. Also to be avoided are beer, wine, coffee, salami, yogurt, chocolate, and any food that is smoked or pickled. These foods and drugs are all fairly common in our culture. Who would have thought that mixing them with an herb could increase blood pressure to dangerous levels, perhaps causing stroke or other significant health problems?

If you are going to take herbs, you must not walk into a shop and take a little of this and a few of those just because you read that they are good for your ailments or your sister said it worked for her. You wouldn't go behind a chemist's counter and help yourself to various pills—and herbs are just as potent, with just as many potential side effects and risks. Please make sure you see a reputable and well-qualified herbalist and disclose all relevant medical information in order to keep yourself safe.

Even if herbs had ever been helpful to me in the past, they were certainly not the answer on the day that I vowed to heal myself. Frustrated by the over-simplified suggestion to try them for my joint problems, I needed far more than that. There was too much wrong with me—and with my life—for an answer as simple as that. The right one had to be out there somewhere; I was just going to have to find it.

I began with the basics, the humble beginning I mentioned earlier. I thought about my body, poor little broken-down machine that it was, worn out like an old car that needed dragging off to the scrap heap. It had been such a long time since I'd been able to be physically active. I missed it. I wanted that back. I wanted those lovely brisk walks. I wanted to dance till my feet hurt. I missed feeling movement in my body.

I thought about Newton's First Law of Motion: an object in

motion stays in motion. I couldn't help but add, *"And an object at rest stays at rest."*

That was it. That was where I had to begin. My body had been at rest far too long.

I had stopped going for walks a few years earlier, mainly because of the returning unstable angina. Without any movement at all, I was so ill as to be high risk for another heart attack. It made sense not to push it by shuffling around the village or the nearby lake like I used to do with great regularity.

Once I'd resolved some significant personal issues that had set off the angina to that terrible place again, my heart settled down. I tried going for walks, but after such a long period of inactivity, my joints were in worse shape than ever. I didn't want to risk enduring the pain and immobility that went with dislocations. So I lived an excessively sedentary life.

I suppose I thought someday I would be in better shape. I didn't know how; I didn't give it much thought. I was too busy putting out fires in my personal life, trying to get through it one day at a time. And at that time, I didn't need any more pain.

Somehow, I had to reconnect with my body. I didn't know what that meant, exactly, but I knew it was where I had to begin if I had any hope of healing myself. I had such a long way to go; the journey ahead seemed more daunting than ever.

But I would not be deterred.

Chapter Six

Affter that awful day at Carburn Park, I realized what I really needed was to start moving again—and then keep moving, even if it was only a little at a time. I'd never truly thought of the human body as a piece of machinery, something mechanical. But really, it is.

Although I hadn't connected this with my many ailments before, I did know one thing: we are not designed to lead sedentary lives. We're built to be physically active. Thousands of years ago there were no machines to do our work for us; our survival depended on movement.

The industrial and technological revolutions have certainly simplified our daily lives, but they've also made it possible for us to do far less than our bodies were designed to do—and we suffer for it. We've become flabby and overweight; our joints and muscles stiffen from lack of use. We pay for this inactivity in countless ways: high blood pressure, increased cholesterol, anxiety, depression, insomnia— the list goes on.

And yet, we all know how much better even a little exercise can make us feel. Those "feel-good" hormones lift our spirits, boost self-esteem, and improve our overall sense of well-being. It's a built-in reward system. We're meant to be active.

Evidence for this is everywhere. The *Daily Mail*'s website, "Mail-Online," ran an article stating that a "couch-potato lifestyle" leaves a man or woman idle, overweight, and eating the wrong foods—and that this is more likely to land someone in hospital than smoking-related diseases. Likewise, *The Daily Telegraph* (Kate Devlin, 26 May 2010) reported that Dr. Richard Weiler, a specialist in sport and exercise medicine, said a lack of fitness is a root cause of more illness than body fat. This includes heart disease, type 2 diabetes, mental health problems, and high blood pressure.

Further, he stated that "cardiorespiratory fitness, which is developed and maintained by regular physical activity, is a better predictor of mortality than obesity."

That made me think about how the human body is rather like a car, which isn't meant to sit still for long periods without being driven. Even a few weeks without running it can leave the battery dead. Leave it for months or years and you'll have to drain old petrol from the tank, replace filters, fluids, spark plugs, coolant—maybe even tires and wheel bearings—before it will work properly again.

Yet, in theory, a well-maintained car can be driven for thousands and thousands of miles without stopping, apart from quick refills of petrol—and the occasional change of driver, of course.

I also thought about the way I approached most things in my life. My tendency was to "go whole hog" and try to run before I could even crawl. Most of the time I managed to pull it off, but physically, that approach was foolish. I knew my body's limitations, but they annoyed me so much that I often ignored them and pushed too hard.

I'd been so disconnected from my body for so many years that it was unreasonable to expect it to do what I demanded. I showed it virtually no compassion or gentleness at all. I wouldn't treat anyone else like that, yet I did it to my very own body all the time.

That's when it hit me: we're a team, my body and I. We're not two separate beings—though for decades I'd acted as though we were.

We had to figure out a way to work together—cooperatively and productively. I had to listen to what it wanted, instead of ignoring it and ordering it around (and then wondering why it ignored me in return).

I understood why a car that had been stationary for years would need special care before it could move again. I wouldn't let a car sit for ten years, then start it up, tear off down the block, and race a Lamborghini—much less expect it to win. Only when I saw my body as a mechanical vehicle, too, did I begin to respect its need for the same careful consideration.

I had always approached life in an all-or-nothing way; everything was black or white. And yet, in so many other areas of life, I'd learned there is grey. That was the key. I just had to find a nice, light shade of grey.

I found it in Tai Chi. I had been interested in it since the late 1980s, but because my personal life constantly exploded in one way or another, I never managed to take classes. Learning Tai Chi from a book was impossible (heaven knows I tried... several times). Eventually, I realized I could get DVDs, which I did while still in England. Surprisingly, although Tai Chi involves slow, gentle movements, it can still give a good workout and even make you break a light sweat. Best of all, it's relaxing and feels like a moving meditation.

This routine had been disrupted during my preparations to move to Canada and afterward, when my daily life had been completely upended. Shortly after arriving in Calgary, I ordered some North American Tai Chi DVDs, knowing my English ones wouldn't work here. I found Scott Cole's "Discover Tai Chi" series online, but with so many adjustments to make, I hadn't tried them yet.

Knowing I needed to reconnect with my physical body, I understood I had to do it carefully and respectfully. I didn't have to run a marathon. I just had to move gently, at a pace my body liked—not one

I wanted, demanded, or forced myself into. I had to do only as much as my body wanted to do.

The less I had been doing in recent years, the less I could do—and the more damage I caused by occasionally diving in and trying to function as I had back when I was in better shape. I had to start small, letting my body—not my stubborn, perfectionistic, "gotta prove how strong I am" determination—be my guide.

After the Carburn Park incident, I didn't dare try walking again right away; the hip pain was still quite bad. From previous experience, I knew it would take a few days to settle. But the following day, I thought I could try the gentle, easy movements of Tai Chi—carefully.

I chose the "AM/PM Workouts" DVD and popped it into the machine. Immediately, I was drawn to Cole's warm spirit, smile, and overall approach. I was especially happy to be reminded of one of Tai Chi's main principles: following the path of least resistance. I had been trying to learn that lesson in other areas of my life for years, and it was particularly helpful in letting go of my "bull in a china shop" approach to getting physically active again.

The AM workout lasted about twelve minutes of gentle, enjoyable movements, followed by a brief "meditation" where he asks you to stand like a tree. He instructs you to feel your energy primarily in your legs and feet, as though rooted to the ground, while your upper body and arms move like branches swaying in the breeze. He suggests applying this principle to life in general: a firmly rooted tree that bends in the wind fares much better than a rigid one.

Standing in my sitting room, eyes closed, I felt my "roots" grounding me while my "branches" stretched and swayed around me. I listened to this lovely man speak. He described energy rising from the ground, flowing into my feet and legs, through the rest of my body, and out my arms and hands. I remembered "tree hugging" and the idea that energy comes up from deep inside the earth through the trunks of trees—and that we can feel it, become part of it, be energized by it. I recalled my acupuncturist from twenty years earlier emphasizing the importance of being outside every day, especially on grass, soil, or sand, to absorb this energy through our feet.

I was reminded of the day my heart problem came roaring back after years of relative calm. Just two weeks earlier my personal life had imploded with a pair of massive emotional shocks, and the stress had left me looking and feeling dreadful. My face was drawn and grey; the strain was obvious. I'd already arranged a trip to Warwick Castle with a friend, and even though I felt awful, I thought maybe the distraction would help. I stuffed several heart remedies into my handbag before we set out.

The castle was beautiful, but I struggled to get through the grounds. My heart simply couldn't keep up. Every step was an effort, and I dragged myself along trying to put on a cheerful face for my friend. Halfway around the grounds, through an old stone archway, I caught sight of the most extraordinary oak tree — the kind of striking, eerie tree you see in films. Its ancient, ivy-covered trunk practically begged me to come closer.

Up to that point, I had never hugged a tree. It had always seemed silly, maybe even embarrassing if anyone was watching. But that day, the tree felt like a giant magnet. I couldn't resist. I went over, wrapped my arms around its trunk and rested my cheek against its rough, enduring bark.

And then it happened: a powerful surge of energy rose up from the ground, into the tree and straight into me. It was beautiful — a tingling rush that made me feel wonderfully alive. I stayed there for several minutes, unable and unwilling to let go. When at last I stepped back, it felt as though the tree had finished with me. I bounced around the rest of the day like a child, full of energy and joy, astonished at what had just happened but grateful for every moment. Later, when friends saw a photo of me taken during my "tree time," they said I looked twenty years younger.

Years later in Calgary, doing Tai Chi in my sitting room, I

thought back to that oak tree. Following Scott Cole's gentle instructions, I swayed like a tree, easily imagining nourishing energy bubbling up from Mother Earth and filling every part of me — because I had *actually felt* that before. With my arms stretching and reaching like branches in the wind, I pictured light streaming down from above, entering the crown of my head. In my mind the two currents — one rising from the ground, one flowing down from the universe — met in my heart. There, they exploded into dazzling light that radiated through my entire body. The experience was so powerful and so moving that it brought me to tears. I was sure some kind of healing had begun, not just in my heart but in every part of me.

Delighted by the results of the AM workout that morning, I tried the PM routine later that evening. It's meant for unwinding and preparing for sleep, but it also works any time you feel stressed. I prefer the soft, warm glow of salt rock lamps around my flat at night — they set the perfect mood for bedtime, meditation, or my evening Tai Chi practice.

Partway through the PM routine is a movement called "Beautiful Woman Turns at the Waist." You place your hands on your kidneys and rotate your upper body in a big circle, first one way, then the other. Scott Cole explains that this movement sends energy to the kidneys. Hearing this thrilled me. I knew it would take more than one exercise to heal my terribly weak kidneys, but at least I had found a place to start.

The PM workout ends with a short meditation. You sit crosslegged and place your palms *down* on your knees — a deliberate difference from the usual palms-up position. Cole explains that according to Tai Chi principles, energy flows out through the palms, and by placing them on your knees you return that energy to the body, letting it circulate in a closed-loop system that nourishes muscles, joints, and every other part of you.

During this brief meditation, the gentle surge of energy I'd felt through the workout continued. When I finished, I switched off the television and moved to the armchair where I always meditate, settling in with my legs crossed, palms still on my knees. Eyes closed, I kept thinking about "energy return." The flow intensified. Most strikingly, I felt it swirling specifically around my kidneys, then into my hips and pelvis, filling these areas with warmth and fullness. I slipped into my usual 20-minute nighttime serenity meditation and, as I did, felt compelled to invite healing white light in through my crown chakra, letting it settle especially in my most troubled areas.

After several minutes the sensation gradually faded, and I went straight to bed. For more than thirty years I had endured terrible hip pain every night, forced to roll over every hour or so or the pain would become excruciating. But not that night. When I woke in the morning I could hardly believe it — no pain. Even the joint pain from my disastrous walk two days earlier had vanished.

I decided to go for a walk. But this time I wasn't the boss. My body would decide the pace and the distance. Every few minutes I'd catch myself slipping into my old autopilot stride, only to slow down again. I wanted to go at least a couple of miles, but my body thought a few blocks was plenty. Twenty minutes later I was back home — and still pain-free.

To say I was elated is an understatement. A slow twenty-minute stroll shouldn't have felt like a triumph for someone who once covered four miles in an hour. But it was a milestone, a true first step. And it turned out to be the beginning of a remarkable and powerful path of self-healing — one that I now share with you.

Chapter Seven

In the days that followed, my body clearly thanked me for letting it exercise on its own terms instead of mine. Respecting its limits and dropping my old "push, push, push" mentality paid off. As long as I remembered that a walk wasn't a race, my body rewarded me with a steady, reasonable pace and, almost immediately, real progress. Tai Chi certainly helped — along with other changes I'll talk about later — but the biggest shift was in recognising that my body and I were a team.

Within days, I noticed improvements in aches and pains I'd carried for years. The severe pain in my lower back was almost gone. I no longer shuffled like a broken old woman, and standing — which had always become excruciating after a short time — was suddenly manageable. Several other nagging troubles had faded too. The gentle movements and energy flow of Tai Chi were turning out to be far more powerful than I'd ever imagined.

A couple of weeks after that first tentative stroll, I woke to a crisp, bright morning and headed out for a walk. I'd already worked my way up to four miles. It wasn't a brisk, head-down march, but it was a good pace nonetheless.

As I walked, I noticed old symptoms flickering back — not like a scolding, but more like a quiet conversation. My body wasn't yelling at me; it was giving me nudges, inviting me to listen.

First to speak was my hip. Impressively, it had taken about two miles before it began to complain. Under my breath, with no one around to hear, I asked it softly what was wrong. The answer that came to me was "fear."

Fear? How could this pain be about fear? What was its purpose? The pain was stopping me from walking — but why would I fear that? I'd always enjoyed walking. What could it represent?

Walking propels us forward. It takes us from one place to another. Could the pain be about moving forward in life? That didn't seem right — moving forward was what I wanted more than anything. I had absolutely no desire to remain stuck where I was. Why would I fear it?

I kept walking and thinking. It was true: I didn't want to stay where I was — renting a flat, living without real security, no "proper" job. I wanted to write books for a living, own a home again, and have enough money to do wonderful things for my family and for people who were suffering and in need. What could be frightening about that?

And then the answer hit me like a bag of bricks. I didn't fear moving forward. I feared trying to move forward and failing. I feared that the future I dreamed of would never come to pass.

For more than forty years, until dementia took her mind, my mother had told me I'd never amount to anything. That I'd never be successful. That I didn't deserve anything good. Intellectually, I knew she was wrong. But deep down, the wounded little girl still believed her. My mother had planted the seeds of her toxic beliefs and fed them until they became poisonous vines, choking the life out of me for decades.

I'd worked long and hard to heal the issues my mother created and had made a lot of progress. But apparently I hadn't yet pulled out those roots completely. Even though she was gone, her words still echoed deep in my soul.

Making matters worse, my life had been in a dreadful sort of limbo for years, which only worsened after moving to Calgary. I didn't feel as though I had anywhere to move toward. I was stuck in a kind of "No Man's Land" — a place where nothing could happen for me, where I'd be trapped in this unmoving, on-hold existence forever. I knew what I wanted, but I had no clue how to get there. Every day felt the same: no progress, no movement, no direction — just more wheel-spinning and getting nowhere.

I wanted desperately to move on but didn't know how. And I feared it never would.

Looking back, I remembered periods when walking hadn't been a problem. After finding that remedy for my heart, I had been unstoppable — four to five miles a day, plus errands, looking after my home and family, and then moving to England, where I continued to be active and busy. My joints hadn't given me too much trouble during those years. How had that been possible?

It made sense now. Homeopathy had cured the emotional roots of my heart trouble. It allowed me to end an unhealthy marriage and make other necessary changes in my life. I was happy. I had a thriving homeopathy practice, a secure financial future, and a modest little home I loved. Life was good, and I was successful. I was helping hundreds of patients feel better, witnessing suffering end, and it thrilled me to be part of that.

Then came England — a life beyond any dream I could have imagined. My days became one grand adventure after another. For nearly six years, I was physically reasonably well by my standards. Sure, I still had headaches, back pain, ongoing poor sleep, kidney issues, and so on, but they were minor compared with the pain and restriction I'd endured from my heart and joint problems.

As I walked through the snow with my slightly grumbling hip, I had an "Aha!" moment. I'd often wondered why my hip pain had eased during those happy years. Now it made perfect sense. I was happy then. Truly happy, for the first time in my life. I had no reason to fear moving forward — or to fear anything about the future. My life was unfolding beautifully, and I was living it.

That was certainly not how I felt now. My body was holding on to this symptom for a reason. To remove it, I first had to acknowledge it — which I did — before imagining it leaving my body. Slowing my pace, I spoke to my hip softly, telling it it was fine, just a little grouchy after so long in stillness. Lovingly, I reminded it that exercise was good for us, and that even if we ached a little at first, we'd be okay.

I added some affirmations, speaking to the issues at hand as I walked. My life was a beautiful adventure. I accepted whatever came. I would flow with events. I looked forward to the future. The statements lifted me. I felt lighter, more positive than I had in a long time.

And then, quite magically, the pain settled. It became barely noticeable. I picked up my pace again — without any problem at all.

As my hip and I made peace, my knee spoke up. The main symptom I'd had with it for 35 years — aside from dislocating — was extreme pain when it bent, which, of course, happens frequently while walking. Even that day, the nature of the pain made me want to keep my leg straight. What was it trying to tell me?

Once again, the answer that came to me was fear. Not surprising — I'd carried fear throughout my life — but what kind of fear was this?

I considered the symptom. A stiff, straight knee that refused to bend could only represent inflexibility. That seemed strange; I've always been adaptable, open-minded, tolerant, and experienced plenty of change. Yet my leg insisted on rigidity. Was there an area of my life where I had become too set in my ways? Maybe I needed to examine those areas and allow myself even more flexibility.

Or was it fear of change? Heaven knew I'd had more than enough of that. Still, there were things I feared would change — and others I feared wouldn't — much like the hip. These symptoms were linked, two perspectives of the same underlying issue. So, I spoke gently to my knee, as I had with my hip, acknowledging the fear and rigidity, reassuring it that movement was safe.

The pain soon eased, and we continued walking.

My lower back had also been grumbling. Over the years, I'd learned that lower back issues often relate to support and security. The base of the spine carries the weight of the upper body, and when we feel unsupported — financially, emotionally, or otherwise — trouble can arise. I'd certainly had my share of financial stress and debilitating back pain over the years. It was time to address it.

Just as I had with the hip and knee, I sent my lower back messages of reassurance. I told it I trusted the universe to provide, repeated affirmations of support, and focused on the present moment. I reminded myself that worrying about next week, next month, or next year was pointless; financial security is fleeting, even for the wealthiest. In that moment, everything was fine. Rent was paid. Food was in the fridge. All was well, right there and then.

With these thoughts and affirmations, my back eased. I was amazed at how quickly and effectively this approach seemed to work. I wondered if it was just coincidence.

About three miles in, my heart began to complain. I was surprised it had waited this long, but then again, I hadn't been moving at a fast pace. It had patiently bided its turn.

As it nudged me, I recalled the conversations we'd had during meditation. My heart had felt "broken" for most of my life, fractured by people, events, and situations — including the wrenching move back to Canada. For years, I'd spoken of heartache in literal terms: "It's like a knife in my heart," "It breaks my heart," and so on. Language shapes the body, and although I'd worked to shift my words, some damage had already been done.

I spoke gently to my heart as I walked, letting it express its pain and "heartache." I wasn't surprised by the emotions that surfaced, but experiencing them while walking that day was different. Tears came, silently expressing what words could not.

I told my heart it was not broken, that it was fine, and merely a storehouse for feelings. I apologized for the burdens it had carried and expressed gratitude for its unwavering work despite past heart attacks and years of unstable angina. I sent it love and healing, visualizing it functioning perfectly, strong and whole.

As we walked together that day — my ailing heart, my joints, and I — I remembered something I had learned years before, when I had briefly "test-driven" being an acupuncture student. According to Chinese medicine, each organ is linked to particular emotions. If an organ is weak, you tend to feel more of its associated emotion. Conversely, if you experience that emotion excessively, the corresponding organ can weaken.

The lungs are tied to grief, which explains why people often develop chest infections or coughs after a significant loss. Anxiety affects the lungs too, sometimes triggering asthma attacks, and can affect the small intestine as well, causing issues like ulcerative colitis.

The kidneys are associated with fear. That resonated with me — I'd lived a life full of fear from the very beginning, and my kidneys were indeed terribly weak. The liver corresponds to anger, and heaven knows I'd swallowed plenty of that over the years, leaving my liver weakened too.

The heart is associated with joy — and therefore, sadness. If there's either too much or too little joy, the heart suffers. I thought about how delighted I was to spend time with my family and friends in Calgary, yet I wasn't feeling much joy about my life overall. Homesickness and sadness weighed heavily on me. I missed Ravenswood desperately — my little fortress of healing and happiness in England. I missed everything and everyone there. Most of the time, I was sad, only uplifted when with loved ones or on the phone to someone back home. I was deeply depressed, doing my best to choke down the pain of this uprooting.

As I walked, I reflected on my chaotic, turbulent life. Joy had always been fleeting. My first years in England had brought happiness, but not without personal and family concerns. Overall, there hadn't been much lasting joy, only little glimpses here and there. If a lack of joy had contributed to my heart trouble, it was no wonder I had been so afflicted in my 30s.

Approaching my home, I focused on connecting with joy. I imagined being with my children, and let that joy fill my heart and circulate through my entire body. A slow smile spread across my face as a fresh energy flowed through me. Repeating to myself how much joy was in my life, my heart symptoms eased, and by the time I reached my flat, I felt wonderful.

Exhausted but elated, I put on soft music and sank into a candlelit bath to reflect on what I'd learned. I had loved the feeling of joy flooding my body, so I returned to it once more — and had one of the biggest "Aha!" moments of my life.

For decades, I had described my life as one long stretch of trauma, stress, and crises. I used to tell people there had never been a time without at least one "movie-worthy" crisis, often several at once. I could pick any month or year and recount the distressing events that had occurred, and people were always stunned. I had said countless times, "All I've ever known is stress and crisis."

It pains me to write that now, but it was true: my life had been turbulent, overloaded with crises and problems. Yet that day, as I focused on filling my body with joy, I suddenly remembered all the joyful moments scattered throughout the chaos. Even as a child, despite the abusive, frightening home environment, there had been moments of joy — not at home, but with friends, neighbours, pets, music lessons, and more.

When I was older, there were the good bits of pregnancies and the thrilling births of my children. In fact, there were millions of wonderful "children" moments and treasures, visits with friends, and funny family stories. There were dinners out, special meals at home, celebrations, laughter — so much joy in my life, even within difficult marriages — yet I had erased every single moment of it every time I said, "All I've ever known is stress and crisis!"

Lying there that day in the bath, it felt as though a lifetime of joy had been dropped on my head all at once, a magical gift. Tears streamed down my face — for once, tears of joy rather than sadness. I embraced every memory, every happy tear, letting the joy wash over and through me. From that day onwards, it became a part of my daily "healing bathing meditation."

As an aside, while doing research for this book, I discovered some fascinating information about the heart in Chinese medicine. The heart can be assaulted by disappointment, criticism, and sexual abuse at a young age — considered one of the greatest betrayals the heart can experience. I had experienced plenty of all of that growing up and into early adulthood. Immediately, I thought about the remedy I had taken so many years ago, the one that had healed my heart for nearly six years.

As I mentioned in Chapter 2, the central theme of that remedy is a feeling of violation, often linked to a history of sexual abuse. It was fascinating to see how Chinese medicine and homeopathy — both powerful "energetic medicines," yet practiced in entirely different ways — connected in this way.

I also understood why that same remedy hadn't worked when my heart problem returned years later. The first time I took it, the cause was ongoing abuse and violation throughout my life, including during that particular marriage. When the symptoms returned, the cause was a broken heart: betrayal, shock, overwhelming grief, and crushing disappointment. There are remedies to address such feelings, but I couldn't find the one that matched the central theme. Remembering the connection to joy, and recognising its presence in my life, seemed to point me in the right direction for healing.

Around this time, I also began experiencing severe hot flushes as menopause approached. They were intense and relentless, occurring every thirty minutes like clockwork. In an instant, I would go from normal body temperature to feeling as if I were on fire, drenched in sweat, especially on my head, neck, and torso. My arms and legs would become clammy and sticky, and I was desperate for water. I needed to peel off layers, hike up skirts or trouser legs — whatever was necessary — and I often felt nauseated if I couldn't cool down immediately.

Minutes later, I would be freezing, grabbing sweaters and blankets, putting on slippers... it was ridiculous. The hot flushes were extremely uncomfortable and mortifying if they happened in front of anyone, and they made sleep almost impossible.

I decided to try my new self-healing technique. First, I needed to understand what the hot flushes were trying to tell me. The rapid swings from hot to cold reflected an imbalance I'd been experiencing for years. I had been striving for a sense of balance in my life: sometimes working too much and not resting or socialising enough, sometimes having too much rest with no work or social interaction. There had been a period in my life when I had just the right balance of work, play, rest, social life, family time, and alone time — and I longed to find it again.

I also had to consider that this was menopause. I'd always appreciated having periods, knowing that women are healthier for them in terms of heart, bones, and other factors. I wasn't saddened by their loss per se; it was just another marker of getting older. And yes, I wasn't thrilled about ageing either. Inside, I often felt like a little kid or my late twenties self, but when I looked in the mirror, I barely recognised the woman staring back — softening, spreading, changing. I felt transplanted into someone else's body, unsure how to relate to it. The hourglass felt as though more sand had shifted to the bottom than the top, and I wasn't happy about it. There was still so much I wanted to do, and I felt I was running out of time.

To address these concerns, I took two actions. First, I made immediate decisions to rebalance how I spent my time. Then I created a set of affirmations to repeat with each hot flush. I told myself that my life and body were in perfect balance, and that I embraced my "wisdom years." I reminded myself that the knowledge and experience I had gained were far more valuable than the youthful, thin body I once had. I acknowledged the positives of this stage of life and chose to view it with acceptance and optimism.

Within a couple of days, the hot flushes slowed to every forty-five minutes. A few days later, they were spaced several hours apart. Within a week, they had almost completely vanished. I was left with only occasional warmth, never uncomfortable, and sometimes a day or two or three would pass between episodes.

To be honest, I was astonished. I hadn't expected such results, especially so quickly. But I realised I had barely dipped my toe into the waters of self-healing. Delightful as the progress was, I had no idea how much more there was to discover — and that it was about to snowball into something truly transformative.

Chapter Eight

Excited about being able to go for walks again with little or no pain, I celebrated reconnecting with my body by thinking about what else I could do for it. I'd long seen myself as a mechanical vehicle — like a car — and that perspective was giving me fresh insight. I didn't want to be a rusted old heap in a scrap yard. I wanted to be a Lamborghini: sleek, powerful, unstoppable. Even if I couldn't imagine ever fully getting there, at least I could try.

I asked myself, if I were a Lamborghini, what would I need to run well and maintain my expensive engine? Fuel, of course. But what kind? There's the cheap stuff, and then there's the high-quality petrol.

Given my financial circumstances at the time, I was doing my best to eat as healthfully as possible on a very skimpy food budget, but it wasn't brilliant. I could barely afford fruits or vegetables, and meat was a luxury. I was eating more rice and pasta than I'd ever eaten in my life, and I wasn't particularly fond of either.

Sure, a car will run on cheap petrol. But engines run on high-quality fuel perform better, last longer, and break down less often.

Repairs cost less, too. And a car can be replaced. Your body cannot. No amount of money will give you a second chance at your one-of-a-kind, irreplaceable self.

Think about it. Would you put cheap petrol in a Lamborghini? Of course not. So why put toxic, artificial, pesticide-laden, fatty, sugary rubbish into your precious body? Just like a car, the human body doesn't thrive long-term on poor-quality food. Additives we can't pronounce, processed foods, junk food, pesticides, too much sugar and fat — they won't give you optimum health. What you put in is what you get out.

Somewhere along the way, I'd stopped eating much tofu or seaweed, and many of the grains, vegetables, and fruits I used to enjoy. Most of what I ate was still relatively healthful, but I'd picked up a few bad habits. I didn't eat enough, often, or consistently. I snuck in some junk food. I drank a couple of glasses of wine most evenings. And for breakfast, an icy glass of Coke had become a daily ritual.

Oddly, I'd started craving chocolate — unusual for someone without much of a sweet tooth. I stuck to bars with nuts or wafers, toning down the sweetness. It was peculiar: I wanted it, but the sweetness was too much to handle, so I limited myself to tiny portions when the craving hit.

And after being disgusted by smoking for most of my life (apart from a few foolish years in my teens), somehow I'd found myself dabbling in my forties, after my heart problem had gone, in an on-again, off-again fashion. I'd spent so much of my life doing the right, healthy thing; this felt like a small rebellion, a way to find balance and be a bit naughty. Honestly, I figured I wasn't going to live long anyway, so what did it matter if I smoked occasionally?

Whatever the reason, the desire was there — a powerful, stubborn urge staring me in the face. Sometimes it made my mouth water; other times, you couldn't have paid me enough to have one.

Moving back to Calgary had largely eliminated these habits — money wasn't there to indulge them. But my shopping trolley still rarely looked particularly nourishing. A few tins of generic soup, a bag of rice, some pasta, a few tomatoes, inexpensive vegetables, maybe some bananas I hated but could afford. I could survive on my meagre budget, but I could not thrive.

Standing in the supermarket queue, I'd watch other people's trollies. Fresh fruit and vegetables piled high, steaks, roasts, chickens, 12-grain bread, cheeses, juices, snacks — so many wonderful, delicious treats. How I longed to walk into a supermarket and buy whatever I wanted, without a thought for the price. It had been a lifelong dream, especially during the financially tight years of single parenting.

In keeping with the idea of putting the best fuel possible into this "Lamborghini wannabe," I wished I could buy organic foods, but the cost was prohibitive. I mentioned this to one of my daughters just after beginning my self-healing mission. She told me about a local farmer's market where many organic items were about the same price as the regular ones — or perhaps just a little more.

I checked it out and she was right. I began buying organic wherever possible. Even some organic meat was around the same price as conventional, but without the added antibiotics, hormones, and other rubbish I didn't want in my body. Soon, I decided it was worth the extra expense to boost my grocery budget and enjoy a less toxic, more varied diet. My body could not function optimally — let alone heal itself — on what I'd been feeding it. Health has no price, and you cannot have good health without a solid starting point.

Of course, diet is only the beginning. I'd heard claims that simply eating a wide range of very healthful, fresh foods — preferably raw or lightly cooked — would be enough to stay well. One source even assured a former cancer patient she would never get cancer again if she just ate the right foods and avoided the wrong ones. Well-meaning, perhaps, but dangerously misleading. As a homeopath, I know that mental and emotional roots often lead to physical symptoms. My research for this book confirmed this countless times: a well-balanced diet alone cannot prevent cancer or other serious illnesses.

Imagine, for instance, a woman in an abusive environment,

surrounded daily by criticism, insults, and resentment, living in a cold, damp house, unable to pursue activities that bring her joy, and chewing over the fear of cancer returning. Or even if her life were otherwise perfect, yet she carried long-standing emotional wounds — I am certain that no diet could keep her cancer-free.

For years, I myself ate an exceptionally healthful diet, rich in whole grains, fruits, and vegetables. I exercised, lived sensibly, did "everything right" — and still developed significant heart disease, not to mention other ailments, including a large mole that began to change shape and colour. Thankfully, it was removed while still dysplastic — one step from malignancy. Left undiscovered, it might have killed me, despite my careful diet.

I also knew a woman who battled breast cancer more than once. She ate a purely organic, highly healthful diet, avoiding refined foods and sugar, yet she lost her fight. Her diet may have helped her fight longer, but it did not address why her body was producing destructive cells in the first place. I've seen similar patterns in many others.

What we eat is crucial, certainly, and can contribute to the quality and length of our lives — but it is far from the only factor. No single element alone can guarantee health, as this book will show.

Once I bit the bullet and increased my grocery budget to include organic foods, I wondered why I hadn't done it years earlier. Money had always been tight — especially during my single-parent years, when even keeping food on the table was a challenge. But there were other times when I could have spent a little more on organic food instead of other, less important things. We always invest our time and money in what matters most.

Having established that this "Lamborghini in training" deserved the highest quality fuel to function at its best, require minimal maintenance, and last as long as possible, the next step was ensuring I used the right kind of fuel for its engine. Put petrol in a diesel engine — or vice versa — and the car will break down, often quickly. If you're lucky, the cost of repairs may be minimal. Depending on your engine, however, it could be catastrophic. Remember: your body is irreplaceable, far more valuable than the most expensive vehicle ever built.

There are a million diets out there, each insisting that their approach to nutrition is the best (and by "diets," I do not mean in the context of weight loss). Some say not to eat fruit within a certain period after vegetables or other foods. Some swear by a vegan diet, others by vegetarian. Some insist that we cannot be completely healthy without eating animal products — and if we do eat them, there are debates about which kinds are best, or worst, for us.

There's the yogi diet, which forbids anything fermented, canned, frozen, jarred, reheated, or leftover, and excludes all animal products apart from organic milk, soft cheese, and butter. Then there are high-protein, low-carb, gluten-free, low-sodium diets. You name it, there are almost as many diets as there are people on the planet, often directly contradicting one another, yet each claiming to be the ultimate solution for our health. I've explored my fair share over decades of ill health.

In the mid-'90s, I first heard about one in particular. A new book, *Eat Right 4 Your Type* by Dr Peter J. D'Adamo, had become "the latest thing." Dr D'Adamo claimed our blood types determine which foods we should eat — or avoid. I thought it was ridiculous, especially when I discovered that my Type "O" supposedly required meat. Because of my ethical stance, I'd rarely eaten animals, so I dismissed the diet immediately, not realising that preferences and principles don't necessarily reflect what our bodies truly need.

Over the years, despite my ethics, I noticed occasional cravings for steak — sometimes to the point of distraction. During a relapse of my heart problem, my vegetarian homeopath in England, Simon, suggested that if I craved beef, I ought to eat it. It wasn't surprising, because one of homeopathy's core principles is that suppression — of symptoms, cravings, or feelings — makes us sick. The body creates symptoms for a reason: to express imbalance, to restore itself, to heal.

Although Simon wouldn't eat beef himself, he advised me to have some regularly because of my craving. I followed his advice, and almost immediately, I felt better — my heart symptoms improved significantly. I honoured the animal with a small prayer of gratitude for giving its life to nourish me, which eased my ethical concerns.

A couple of years before starting this self-healing journey, I revisited the blood type diet. I'm not entirely sure what prompted it, though I suspect my persistent craving for beef triggered the memory of Type O people needing meat. Curiosity won out. I was stunned to discover that the diet had existed since the 1950s and was well known in Japan, where people are sometimes asked their blood type at job interviews. Each type is associated with particular personality traits, susceptibility to illnesses, responses to stress, and suitable activities. It made sense that employers might find this useful when matching candidates to roles — though I still couldn't see how blood type could determine diet or personality.

The key lies in the antigens that make each blood type distinct. Blood Type A has the A antigen, Type B has B, Type AB has both, and Type O has neither. Along with the Rh factor (positive or negative), these antigens determine blood compatibility. For instance, giving Type A blood to a Type O person triggers an immune attack on the red blood cells, which can be fatal.

According to Dr D'Adamo, proteins in foods called lectins react with our blood type antigens. Eating foods incompatible with your blood type can cause clumping of blood cells in certain organs or systems, leading to disease, pain, or dysfunction. Most lectins are eliminated, but around 5% enter the bloodstream, triggering various reactions. Each blood type has foods deemed "medicinal," "allowed," or "poison." Beef, for Type O, is considered "medicinal," explaining my overwhelming cravings during periods of illness. My body knew what it needed and wouldn't relent until it got it.

Many diets advise limiting red meat, but for Type O people — the majority — beef, venison, lamb, and mutton are medicinal and should be eaten regularly. Foods like wheat, coconut, coffee, black tea, and potatoes are considered "poison," and wheat in particular can interfere with insulin and slow metabolism, leading to weight gain. Now I understood why those foods always left me feeling heavy, sluggish, and depleted.

Some "poison" foods I didn't much like anyway, but others I loved — sweetcorn, melons, rhubarb, lentils. Still, fed up with being ill, I figured I had nothing to lose — and much to gain — by trying this diet.

Since adopting the blood type diet, I've strayed occasionally, then returned, always with the same results. I am not one to follow trends; I prefer to "do my own thing." Yet following this diet has been among the most beneficial things I've done. I feel lighter, more energetic, and mentally sharper. My former sluggishness disappears, and I am far more productive.

Having proven that the blood type diet significantly improves how I feel, I try not to put diesel in my petrol engine anymore. When I feed my body the fuel it is designed for, it rewards me by functioning efficiently on every level. The diet doesn't solve everything, but it makes me feel far better and has become an important piece of the self-healing puzzle.

And as I contemplated the consequences of putting diesel in a petrol engine, I faced a subject I'd known about for thirty years but had not fully addressed. I recognised it as the next piece of the puzzle — one that it was time to put into place.

Chapter Nine

As I looked at nutrition, I knew I had to do something about getting enough calcium. It is absolutely essential for various processes in the human body, including heart function, yet I don't believe we should rely on cow's milk for it. How can cow's milk be considered an essential part of our diet when its purpose is to feed calves until they are old enough to be weaned? How does it make any sense that humans are supposed to drink it? Just because it has been consumed for centuries doesn't make it rational or beneficial; it simply means it was available and eventually became an accepted part of our diet.

Essential? Not on your life. Good for you? No way. Talk about putting diesel in a car that requires petrol. At least diesel and petrol operate similar engines. But giving cow's milk to a human is like putting orange juice in the petrol tank. Our bodies simply aren't designed to tolerate it — it was made for a species with four stomachs. Consuming it is a terrible assault on a body ill-equipped to process it.

It's no surprise that cow's milk is the most common food allergen in North America. Because the symptoms are often subtle, it's frequently overlooked. Reactions vary from person to person but can include fatigue, headaches, hyperactivity, runny nose, nasal congestion, frequent colds, chest infections, asthma, ear infections, vomiting, diarrhoea, eczema, hives, trouble sleeping, and even bed-wetting. Consider how common these ailments are, especially in children. Even breastfed babies whose mothers consume cow's milk may experience nappy rash, eczema, or digestive discomfort.

Constantly bombarding the body with a food allergen is asking for trouble, and there is a wealth of research to back this up. For instance, in *Discover Magazine* (August 2000), Dr T. Colin Campbell, PhD, a renowned nutritional biochemist at Cornell University, revealed how cow's milk can contribute to chronic illness. Growing up on a dairy farm, he had firmly believed milk was essential to health — but his research proved otherwise.

After years of study, he concluded that it is "unnatural" for humans to drink milk or consume milk products. The Physicians Committee for Responsible Medicine (PCRM), a Washington, DC-based non-profit with over 100,000 members, promotes preventive medicine and high ethical standards, and opposes consumption of cow's milk in any form.

Firstly, they point out that milk is a poor source of calcium for humans — no surprise, since it wasn't intended for us. Neal Barnard, head of PCRM, states, "It would be hard to imagine a worse vehicle for delivering calcium to the human body." Secondly, the health risks associated with milk are alarming. Most people in Asia, Africa, southern Europe, and Latin America have difficulty digesting lactose, the main sugar in milk. Cow's milk has also been found to stimulate growth hormones in humans, increasing the risk of being overweight and developing various diseases.

Research shows that milk does not build strong bones in humans; in fact, it can do more harm than good. While recent studies suggest we may need less calcium than once thought, we need better-quality calcium than that found in cow's milk. Good sources include eggs, sardines, broccoli, leafy vegetables, tofu, salmon, molasses, baked beans, peas, dried beans, parsnips, artichokes, almonds, peanuts, walnuts, sesame seeds, and sunflower seeds. This is not an exhaustive list — and there's also the option of making soup with the bones of animals or birds, which, according to a Chinese doctor I consulted many years ago, produces an excellent calcium-rich broth.

Since 1965, studies have shown a strong link between milk consumption and several types of cancer, including liver cancer and two increasingly common cancers in Europe and North America: breast and prostate. Yet in Asia, where most people do not consume milk products, breast cancer is rare. A 1989 study revealed that in Scandinavia and the Netherlands, where milk consumption is high, breast cancer rates are also high. Similarly, worldwide research into prostate cancer shows it is far more prevalent where dairy products are consumed than where they are not.

What shocked me most was the link between dairy consumption and hip fractures. Worldwide studies show that the more dairy people consume, the more susceptible they are to broken hips. In North America and Northern Europe, where dairy consumption is two to three times higher than in Asia and Africa, fracture rates are also two to three times higher. A 12-year Harvard Nurses' Health Study produced similar results.

To make matters worse, many commercial dairy farmers are known to give cows synthetic growth hormones and antibiotics, which can end up in the milk we drink. Regulations vary from country to country, so depending on where you live, you may be more or less susceptible to these risks.

Adding to the concern, the natural lifespan of a dairy cow has been reduced from around 25 years to a mere five. During that time, she is forced into constant milk production, which exhausts her body and weakens her immune system. This makes her prone to mastitis, a painful infection of the udder. If the infection goes undetected, her milk may contain blood or pus, and antibiotics may be added if she is returned to milking too soon.

On the website of the Arizona Center for Advanced Medicine, Dr Samuel S. Epstein, author of *What's In Your Milk*, explains:

"rBGH (recombinant Bovine Growth Hormone) is a genetically engineered, potent variant of the natural growth hormone produced by cows." He notes that it increases milk production by around 10% and, although said to be safe for consumers, this is "blatantly false."

Dr Epstein states that rBGH makes cows sick and causes roughly 20 toxic effects, including mastitis. He adds, "rBGH milk is chemically and nutritionally different from natural milk." Even more concerning, rBGH increases levels of Insulin-Like Growth Factor (IGF-1), which promotes cell division in humans. According to his research, "Excess levels of IGF-1 have been incriminated as a cause of breast, colon and prostate cancers."

Dr Epstein's book "...presents [his] trailblazing scientific publications since 1989, which have played a major role in influencing other nations...to ban rBGH milk."

With so much research warning against cow's milk consumption, I could go on at length, but this is enough to make the point clear.

However, I needed calcium, one of the most important and necessary minerals for the human body. Not only does it help with blood clotting, sending and receiving nerve signals, and releasing hormones and other chemicals, it is essential for the squeezing and relaxing of muscles — including the heart, which relies on calcium to beat and relax properly.

Over the years, through my health studies and especially my deep dive into the heart, I'd learned that unlike most cells in the body, heart muscle cells do not regenerate. All available information insisted we die with the same heart cells we were born with. Once those cells are deprived of blood (and therefore oxygen) during a heart attack, they're gone. The scarring left behind causes extra strain on the heart and increases the risk of further heart attacks or heart failure.

Given all the damage my heart had endured over the years of frequent oxygen deprivation, I knew I had to do everything possible to help what was left of it function as well as it could. And if I was really lucky, maybe I could even prolong my life a few years — especially if I could improve my overall health. After decades of dead-ends and failed attempts, my self-healing project was my last chance. Honestly, I wasn't holding my breath for more than a little improvement.

Rededicating myself to wellness, I considered my heart's calcium needs. I remembered something I used to get from my Calgary acupuncturist, Dr Alison Jiang: mineral whey powder made from goat's milk. Just a couple of tablespoons in a cup of boiling water made a delicious, nourishing drink. Containing more than 20 naturally occurring minerals — including phosphorus, magnesium, iron, copper, zinc, manganese, and potassium — it was an excellent calcium source. It had almost no protein and came from free-range goats whose food was free of pesticides, herbicides, growth hormones, and antibiotics.

Although Alison and I had been friendly nearly two decades earlier, I hadn't seen her since before I moved to England. I thought it would be fun to drop by her office, say hello, and buy some mineral whey. Her office was near my flat, so I popped by a few times, but found it empty. Weeks passed. Meanwhile, I carried on with my self-healing project, eventually giving up on getting it from Alison and ordering it online instead.

Everything happens for a reason and in its own time. As it turned out, I was destined to meet Alison again, but not for several months. That meeting would reveal why I hadn't met her sooner — because if I had, I might have rejected some of the most fascinating, life-giving, even life-saving information I would ever hear. I would have missed removing a major stumbling block to my healing and discovering one simple fact that gave me more hope than I'd had in years.

But that piece of the puzzle wasn't ready yet. In the meantime, the next revelation was startling. Frightening, even. I prayed it wasn't too late to undo a lifetime of damage — damage caused, ironically, by a process that keeps us alive.

Chapter Ten

In the midst of doing research for this book, a very dear friend in India mentioned a book by Ray Strand, MD called *What Your Doctor Doesn't Know About Nutritional Medicine May Be Killing You*. Strangely, this was just the sort of book that I would not normally be interested in reading at all. But a little voice inside urged me get it right away. I did, having learned (very much the hard way) that that little voice is always right.

I was intrigued to discover that this book fit perfectly as the next - and very powerful - piece of the self-healing puzzle. With the car analogy helping me to reconnect with what my body needed in a physical, mechanical way, this book provided relevant information that was nothing short of sobering.

Dr. Strand begins by explaining that in the early 1900s, most people died of infectious diseases such as pneumonia, TB, diphtheria and influenza with the average life expectancy being a mere 43 years old. In the latter half of the last century, and continuing into the present one, the ongoing development of antibiotics has changed all of that. Instead of dying young from infectious diseases, we were - and are - primarily suffering and dying from degenerative diseases that sometimes begin at relatively early ages. These include coronary artery disease, arthritis, macular degeneration, cancer, Alzheimer's, Parkinson's disease and MS but there are many, many more. These and other degenerative diseases are caused by oxidative stress and a lack of cellular nutrition.

I will discuss cells in greater detail in later chapters but for the moment, I want to stick to the basic mechanics of the body and some of its most essential requirements. Among them are specific nutrients that we simply cannot get in large enough quantities just from eating a well-balanced diet, yet they are necessary for us to be well.

In the interests of brevity and clarity, please bear with me while I give you a ridiculously oversimplified explanation of an extremely complex process. I've got a lot of ground to cover in this book. We need to see the whole forest; I do not want to get bogged down in looking at every leaf on the individual trees.

All cells contain mitochondria, microscopic organisms that are the "power houses" where chemical energy is stored for later use. First, carbohydrates, fats and proteins are broken down by processes within the cell (this is called metabolism). These nutrients contain chemical energy, which is trapped and stored by forming ATP (adenosine triphosphate) molecules. ATP becomes a sort of energy "currency" and is used by our cells to carry out their various tasks.

During the production of ATP, the mitochondria reduce oxygen by transferring electrons. Most of the time, this does not present a problem. But occasionally, an electron is not paired with another, resulting in an oxygen molecule with at least one unpaired electron in its outer orbit.

These molecules are called "free radicals". It was many years ago that I first heard some rumblings about free radicals and thought 'Yeah, right, blah blah blah, what's the big deal?' I wish I'd paid attention, for they are a very big deal, indeed. They carry a relatively strong electrical charge and need to be neutralised quickly. Otherwise, they can create even more free radicals, causing damage to the part or parts of the body where they occur. They damage cell membranes, proteins, even the DNA in the nucleus. This damage is called oxidative stress, and it is the cause of numerous degenerative diseases, such as the ones listed above.

Yes, it's scary, isn't it? But there is help in the form of antioxidants.

An antioxidant is any substance that can give up an electron to the unpaired free radical, thereby neutralising it before it can do any damage. We are capable of producing some antioxidants, such as dismutase, catalase, and glutathione peroxidase. But we do not produce all of the necessary antioxidants we require, nor do we produce a large enough quantity. We must get the rest from our food, and more importantly, from supplements because it is the only way to get the correct amounts.

Now before I go any further, I have to say that I used to think people who took supplements were being foolish and wasting their money. I figured that most of us keep getting by just fine without gulping a load of pills, and besides, it was so confusing, with this person saying you need this and that and a couple of those, and someone else saying you need some other new and exciting weird little enzyme or mineral or whatever. But of course, people are still getting sick. Degenerative diseases are everywhere, to one extent or another. So apparently, we haven't been "getting by just fine."

It is well past time for us to consider prevention of illness, rather than waiting until it's too late and hoping there will be a cure or treatment available.

Dr Strand admits to having been one of those people who thought supplements were unnecessary. But to cut a long story short (he did write a whole book on the subject, after all), after an "up close and personal" experience, he changed his tune. His wife had been ill for many years. As time went on, she took more and more medications, but instead of getting better, she developed more symptoms and became even sicker. Eventually, a friend introduced her to the concept of supplements, and she decided to give them a try.

Her recovery was remarkable and Dr Strand determined to discover more about the subject. Surprised and most impressed by what he learned, in time, he incorporated this knowledge into his medical practice and began using it to help his patients. His book provides loads of evidence and case histories of the dramatic improvements he has witnessed, along with details about why specific supplements were helpful in particular conditions.

With oxidative stress being the cause of so much of our suffering, it is a blessing to discover a relatively simple way to help prevent it. A thorough look at this topic is beyond the scope of this book; however, it is essential that I introduce you to it as a part of the self-healing puzzle.

Most antioxidants come from fruits and vegetables, with the most common being Vitamins C, E and A, and beta-carotene. There are others, such as coenzyme Q_{10} (ubiquinone, otherwise known as CoQ_{10}) and alpha-lipoic acid. Each one has a specific job and all of them work together to clean up the destructive free radicals that roam through our bodies. For example, Vitamin C is water-soluble so it works best to neutralise free radicals in blood and plasma, whereas Vitamin E is fat-soluble and works best within cell membranes. It actually attaches itself to the LDL or "bad" cholesterol, thereby making it much less harmful. The point is to have many and varied antioxidants to give ourselves the best possible defense against dangerous free radicals.

In order to do their job, antioxidants need many other nutrients such as copper, selenium, zinc, folic acid and some of the B vitamins. We are constantly producing free radicals as a byproduct of metabolism; there is no way to stop this occurring. All we can do is reduce or eliminate them as quickly as possible so they do not have a chance to cause any oxidative damage in our bodies, and we do this by ensuring that we've got an adequate clean-up crew.

There have been numerous studies of CoQ_{10} since it was first discovered in 1957 in the mitochondria of a cow's heart. Eventually, normal blood levels of CoQ10 were established in humans, later providing us with a clear link between the severity of heart failure and diminished levels of this powerful and energy-producing enzyme. Further to this startling revelation, significantly decreased amounts of it have been discovered in patients with diabetes, periodontal disease, cancer and heart disease, with the most clearly established deficiencies seen in people with congestive heart failure and cardiomyopathy.

CoQ10 is not only one of the most powerful antioxidants in the war against free radicals but its most important role is to help create energy. It is found in trace amounts in certain foods, such as organ meats, sardines and peanuts and the body can manufacture it, but it is a very complicated process and requires several specific vitamins and minerals. Missing any one detail can prevent its production entirely.

Another supplement that Dr Strand has found to be extremely powerful and helpful for many of his patients is grape-seed extract. It is a bioflavanoid antioxidant, thousands of which are found in our fruits and vegetables. With brilliant anti-inflammatory properties, in high enough doses these antioxidants can reduce or eliminate all sorts of symptoms. In terms of easing or preventing chronic inflammatory diseases (one of which is cardiovascular disease), grape-seed extract is thought to be the best of the bioflavanoid antioxidants.

Speaking of inflammatory diseases, the suffix, "-itis", means "inflammation." From having begun studies as a master herbalist some years back, I know that ginger root is an amazing anti-inflammatory, and with the correct dosage relieves or eliminates virtually any minor ailment such as sinusitis, arthritis, bursitis, myofasciitis etc. Therefore, I would think that grape-seed extract, with its anti-inflammatory properties, would also relieve, eliminate or prevent these and other "-itis" ailments, as well. Such benefits, along with its other antioxidant activity with regard to preventing or treating degenerative diseases, make it one of the most important supplements that we can take.

Although a moderate exercise program is an essential component of a healthy lifestyle, Dr Strand points out that people who exercise excessively show signs of oxidative damage. This explains why sometimes, people who seem to be very health-conscious and exercise at length every day may develop heart disease, cancer and so on. Those people who have to be very active, such as professional athletes, should be sure to take adequate supplements in an effort to reduce the free radical damage to their bodies before it makes them critically ill.

Long-term stress is another major cause of oxidative stress. With an exceptionally crisis-filled, stressful life going right back to my birth, when I read these words the enormity of them hit me as though I'd been kicked in the stomach. In an instant, fear flooded through my veins like so much ice water. I could see why I had developed a heart problem in my 30s, and wondered what other nastiness might be lurking, waiting to be discovered within my banged up, stressed-out, neglected old body.

I thought about my particular concerns and made note of the specific nutrients that were relevant, such as CoQ10, grape-seed extract, Vitamins E, B, C and more. I checked Dr Strand's recommended dosages and read the sections on possible risks, side effects, interactions etc. Just to be sure, I checked several other sources, too, before deciding on the supplements I thought were most suitable and necessary for my situation, and off I went to buy them.

Dr Strand says repeatedly that although nutritional supplements can dramatically reduce or even eliminate symptoms, they do not "cure" diseases. This makes perfect sense to me, because in all likelihood, even if the symptoms had been removed, my guess is that if patients stopped taking the supplements, the symptoms would return because the original reason for them would still be present (and which is why I wrote this book, and is precisely what later chapters will address).

Whether or not that is the case, there is not one specific "something" that can cure everything all by itself. Not "the ultimate diet", not one particular healing modality, not a specific exercise regimen. There are many pieces to the magnificent healing puzzle, each of which plays its own significant role, and all of which, when combined, create one fairly logical, understandable, and simple, yet powerful picture.

Nonetheless, the information contained in Dr Strand's book is one of the most important pieces of that puzzle. I recommend his book wholeheartedly as a place to begin if you're looking for a balanced and sensible source of information about nutritional supplements that could make a world of difference on your self-healing journey.

It was shortly after this that I stumbled upon a huge piece of this puzzle that was so incredible, so shocking and so life-changing that there were simply no words. Its roots lie in a Nobel-prize-winning bit of information that few people know about, yet it revolutionises health care, with the potential to save millions of lives each year, and vastly improve the quality of the lives of many more.

Chapter Eleven

I n the months following my many failed attempts to contact Alison Jiang, my former acupuncturist, I could not get her out of my head. Although I was preoccupied with many aspects of this self-healing project and my work, every now and then I tried again to reach her by phone until eventually, I was successful. After a brief catch-up, we arranged a meeting for the following afternoon. It would prove to be a meeting that gave me more hope than I think I'd ever had. It was a meeting that changed my life. And what I learned can change yours, too.

Looking back, it would appear as though the universe did not want me to meet with Alison until I was ready to receive the information she would give me because it has proven to be a significant part of this self-healing project, as you will soon see.

I began to tell her about my self-healing project and excitedly, she told me about a nutritional supplement that she had been taking for 16 months. Prior to reading Dr Strand's book, which I had just barely finished when Alison and I met that day, I would have smiled and nodded, whilst completely disregarding the notion of a supplement. Instead, I asked her to tell me more.

A cardiology specialist in China before coming to Alberta many years ago, Alison's professional opinion was most valuable. With another of her specialties being in the area of diet and nutrition, I was even more convinced that I ought to hear her out. She urged me to try this product, ProArgi-9+™, mainly because of my ongoing heart and kidney problems, but she said it helps all manner of ailments.

She told me about the developer of this product, Dr Joseph Prendergast, who had been giving it to his patients and in 19 years had not had one single admission to hospital for any sort of cardiovascular problem. Not one heart attack, not one stroke, not one stent, not one bypass operation.

This is especially impressive, given that as an endocrinologist, 80% of his practice consists of diabetics, which makes them high risk for heart attack and stroke. Prior to using this product, on average of 30% of Dr Prendergast's patients were admitted to hospital each year. He used to refer many of his patients to three cardiologists in his town, but all three of their businesses dried up and they had to move away after Dr Prendergast's concoction made such a significant improvement in his patients' health.

Alison told me, too, that ProArgi-9+ had been responsible for people coming off heart and kidney transplant lists, and for making them far healthier than they had been in some time. She sent me home with some of this intriguing powder and a couple of DVDs about it. Eager to learn more, I settled in to watch them that evening — but not without first dissolving one scoop of this curious powder in a glass of water so I could sip its citrus goodness whilst learning all about it.

What I learned was so impressive, I could not take my eyes off the television, and to be honest, what I learned was so powerful, I wept tears of hope and joy. With thousands of studies and mountains of medical and scientific research to support the claims about this product, I couldn't wait to give it a try.

So what is it and how does it work?

To answer these questions in detail would require several chapters but I am excited to give you the highlights of what I've learned. We begin with the men who were awarded the 1998 Nobel Prize in Physiology or Medicine, Robert Furchgott, Louis Ignarro and Ferid Murad, for their discoveries regarding the role nitric oxide plays in the cardiovascular system. It has been called "the miracle molecule" and "the spark of life" because it is extraordinarily important in the functioning and health of every cell in the body. In recent decades, growing research about nitric oxide indicates that it may both prevent and cure numerous diseases, which, as you will see from its history, is actually quite shocking.

Outside the body, it is toxic, an environmental pollutant that is found in car exhaust and smog. When discharged from power plants, nitric oxide reacts with oxygen and creates nitrogen dioxide, which is responsible for "acid rain". It is also extremely reactive inside the body, and can become a dangerous free radical, which we know is not only the leading cause of aging, but also numerous degenerative diseases, as discussed in the previous chapter.

Alfred Nobel invented dynamite, an explosive made from nitroglycerin. Its derivative, nitric oxide, was found to be a useful drug for various ailments. Plagued by ill health throughout much of his life, one of Nobel's main complaints was angina. In a letter to colleague Ragnar Sohlman dated October 25, 1896, he wrote, "My heart trouble will keep me here in Paris for another few days at least, until my doctors are in complete agreement about my immediate treatment. Isn't it the irony of fate that I have been prescribed (nitroglycerine) to be taken internally! They call it Trinitrin, so as not to scare the chemist and the public." (*The Legacy of Alfred Nobel*, R. Sohlman, The Bodley Head Ltd. London, 1983)

Nitroglycerin has been widely used in the treatment of angina to prevent heart attacks for more than 100 years without anyone understanding how it worked. Finally, after years of research Furchgott, Ignarro and Murad, who share the Nobel prize in Physiology or Medicine for 1998, discovered that it acts by releasing nitric oxide. This gas is released in the endothelium, being the innermost layer of cells that line the blood vessels, and it diffuses through to the smooth muscle cells, causing them to relax. This widens the blood vessels, causing increased blood flow, improved circulation and oxygen to the heart muscle, and reducing the likelihood of heart attack.

Dr Louis Ignarro has published numerous articles and books related to his research on the subject of nitric oxide. One of his books is entitled *No More Heart Disease: How Nitric Oxide Can Prevent - Even Reverse - Heart Disease and Strokes*. His research into nitric oxide, as well as that of his fellow Nobel prize-winners, led to Dr John P Cooke, MD, PhD, writing *The Cardiovascular Cure: How to Strengthen Your Self Defense Against Heart Attack and Stroke*. Truly, the nitric oxide connection to curing and preventing cardiovascular disease has been one of the most significant medical discoveries of all time.

Nitric oxide is synthesised by an enzyme called nitric oxide synthase, and is necessary for virtually all of your cells if you're going to be well. In 1992, scientists voted nitric oxide "molecule of the year", understanding that it plays a significant role as a chemical messenger between nerves and cells. It has been proven that tiny amounts of nitric oxide are essential for normal functioning of the immune system, the liver, pancreas, uterus, gastrointestinal system, cardiovascular system, reproductive organs, lungs, the brain, memory, and so much more. It has also been proven to aid in fertility and sexual function in both men and women, and led to the creation of Viagra.

To think that as recently as the 1980s, it was simply seen as just another toxic chemical, when in fact, it is vital to the healthy functioning of virtually every aspect of the human body; this is truly incredible.

No doubt Alfred Nobel would have loved to hear this. Not long before his death in 1896, he established the Nobel Peace Prize apparently due to his regret about creating destructive explosives that were used regularly in war.

Nitric acid acts on the lining of the blood vessels, working to keep them smooth like teflon, instead of sticky like velcro. In theory, this should make it virtually impossible for plaque to stick and create atherosclerosis. It should also make it impossible for platelets to gather and form blood clots.

However, although the human body creates nitric oxide (with the help of a semi-essential amino acid called L-arginine), it does not create enough of it to undo the damage caused by troublemakers such as free radicals, high blood pressure, high sugar levels and cholesterol.

Cardiologist Dwight Lundell, MD, says these are amongst the many factors that cause an inflammatory response in the blood vessels, which is the body's defense against just such attacks. That inflammatory response is meant to fight off bacteria, viruses, foreign invaders. Under normal circumstances, the body can cope with these temporary situations and the inflammation disappears. However, when we expose ourselves to repeated injury by products that the body was never meant to process, such as additives and chemicals, this ongoing assault creates a chronic inflammatory process that leads to cardiovascular disease, obesity and diabetes.

Imagine if you were to brush your skin hard several times a day, every day, it would be painful, bleeding and raw. If you carried on doing this for years, can you imagine the state of your skin? The infection, the pain, the swelling, the scarring... This is essentially what happens to the inside of your blood vessels with repeated expo-sure to harmful substances (especially, for example, with smoking). Dr Lundell says that he has seen this kind of inflammation inside the arteries of 5,000 patients, and that it is this, and not cholesterol, that causes cardiovascular disease. When there is no inflammation, cholesterol moves freely through the bloodstream, causing no trouble whatsoever. But it becomes trapped in the lining of inflamed blood vessels.

Further, Dr Lundell says that the worst culprits for setting up this inflammatory process are sugar, flour and all products made from them, as well as the excessive consumption of omega-6 vegetable oils, such as soybean, corn and sunflower. Another major contributor is being overweight, as fat cells pour out large quantities of inflammation-producing chemicals.

We can lessen the inflammation to some extent by limiting our intake of known foods or other products that will create a problem, but there are many factors that we cannot control, such as environmental toxins, pollutants, or the inflammation that is created as a result of processes within the body when we are under stress. There is no way our bodies can produce enough L-arginine, and therefore enough nitric oxide, to undo this kind of damage.

People sometimes buy L-arginine as a supplement by itself, but on its own, it can actually do more harm than good. Or it may do no good at all, as its action as a pure enzyme is usually very brief. It needs to be combined with another amino acid, L-citrulline, which draws out the action of L-arginine. ProArgi-9+ contains L-arginine, L-citrulline and more. It took Dr Prendergast, or "Dr Joe", as he likes to be called, 15 years to perfect the specific combination of ingredients and their dosages in this product.

One of the best parts of the DVDs that Alison loaned me about ProArgi-9+ was the lengthy interview with the unassuming and likable Dr. Joe.

Let me introduce you to him. A graduate of Wayne State University in Detroit in the 1960s, he began his residency at Henry Ford Hospital, achieving the position of Chief Resident for two years before moving to California. He became a Research Fellow at the Metabolic Research Unit, University of California Medical Center in San Francisco.

For many years he was an internist and endocrinologist, eventually setting up his own practice with a specialty in endocrinology. From 1970 to the time of this writing, he has been a staff physician at Stanford Hospital. He is the president of the non-profit Pacific Medical Research Foundation, which he created in 1986. On his CV, there is an extensive list of positions he holds, detailing President of this and Director of that, all to do with endocrinology, diabetes, internal medicine, metabolism and so on.

Dr Joe has published numerous medical articles in well-known publications such as the American Journal of Medicine, and the New England Journal of Medicine and Diabetes Care. To say that he is well respected in the medical community is an enormous understatement.

Dr Joe had occasion to undergo an abdominal CT scan many years ago, at the tender age of 37. He was stunned to discover that his blood vessels were loaded with plaque and atherosclerosis, like those of an 85-year-old man. With his father having died of heart disease in his 50s, Dr Joe did not want to follow in those footsteps. Already an athlete with a healthy diet and lifestyle, he was determined to discover whether there might be anything else he could do to improve his situation.

So began his research into the causes and possible cures or treatments for cardiovascular disease, which ultimately led him to the combination of products that he began using on himself and his patients in 1991. As above-mentioned, almost immediately, he stopped admitting patients to hospital for cardiovascular complaints because quite simply, they stopped having any.

Twenty-five years after that first and frightening CT scan, he had another one for an unrelated concern. The doctor who examined the first test just happened to be examining the second one, too. He looked at Dr Joe and said, "How did you do it?" Every trace of the atherosclerosis was gone. Now, in his 70s, he is said to have the vascular system of a 15-year-old.

According to available information about ProArgi-9+, its powerful antioxidant and anti-inflammatory benefits could make it possible to prevent or treat a multitude of illnesses, including cancer, and a wide range of degenerative diseases. It is also said to reverse the aging process, with claims that it sets body clocks back 20 years or more.

It does not work overnight; it is said to take several weeks to begin to notice improvements, and Dr Joe guesses it can take 1-2 years to feel the full effect of it, depending on a person's circumstances. I suppose this makes sense. After all, we don't become chronically ill overnight; it takes years. Although we love immediate results, faster internet, speedier service, and pills that work NOW, we must leave our need for instant gratification at the door and learn to be more patient.

Personally, after a week to ten days taking four scoops of ProArgi-9+ a day, I noticed an improvement in my overall energy. Despite short nights that would have had me dragging through my days, I was more alert and productive than usual. At just under three weeks, I remember being out for my morning walk, burning along as fast as I could possibly go when I noticed that I felt strong - physically strong and energised, with a sense of muscular power that is difficult to describe. It was incredible! I suppose I may have felt like that as a child; I don't know. I just know I had not felt like that in at least the last few decades and it was absolutely marvellous.

In those early weeks, my colour improved and my eyes looked brighter. People were beginning to comment on the fact that I looked healthier. Within six weeks, they were saying I looked younger, that I was radiant, and that even my hair looked healthier. I felt as though I had been lit up from the inside, energised by this product and it was beginning to show. It gave me hope that there was already dramatic improvement taking place in my heart, my blood vessels, in every cell in my body. It wasn't long before I decided to become a distributor for this amazing product, which is now sold in more than 30 countries around the world.

I was especially excited to learn that I could improve my cardio-vascular health more than I had ever thought possible, but there was still that nagging bit of knowledge in my head about "dead tissue" and scarring due to heart attack damage. It was also a well-known fact that muscle cells do not regenerate in the body, which of course includes the heart. I had read loads of literature about the heart during the many years of my illness and all of it gave the same bad news.

As much as I liked to envision my heart being perfectly healed and well and had been doing this down the years during the odd meditation, there was always that little voice in my head, taunting me with "You know that's impossible." I had to agree with it, so I continued to have thoughts about the dead scar tissue, and the fact that my heart had sustained an awful lot of damage and was not very functional. To tell myself anything else made me feel like a liar.

I thought that at best, this product could give me several more years, especially combined with everything else I was doing toward self-healing. I hoped that it might strengthen what was left of my heart but I felt overwhelming sadness about the damage never being healed, and likely shortening my life considerably.

It was then that I made a startling discovery, and it was a discovery that changed everything.

Alison had given me a pamphlet about ProArgi-9+, which I'd put on my desk on arriving back home. After watching the DVDs, I was convinced of the product's ability to vastly improve the health of anyone who takes it but still, I wanted to do a little research of my own.

One of the ingredients in ProArgi-9+ is D-ribose, and I was most excited to discover that it energises the heart. Produced by the body, it is connected with the production of ATP (adenosine triphosphate), which you may recall from Chapter 10 is the fuel that our cells create from the nutrients we consume, and it is then stored in the mitochondria, the power storage units in our cells.

D-ribose is an important component of a cardiac rejuvenation regimen and when administered to patients having certain kinds of heart surgery (especially up to an hour of forced cardiac arrest during bypass surgery), there is significant improvement in heart muscle function afterward, as compared with those who do not get it. Further, the amount of improvement is directly related to the amount of ATP in the heart muscle.

This is another one of those enormous topics and I do not want to get bogged down in details, but rather, just give you the most important bits.

As I read the Life Extension Magazine website's information on D-ribose, I saw this: "Ischemic (no blood flow) events such as heart attack can cause areas of the heart muscle to 'hibernate' exactly as if they were awaiting a higher-energy environment to return to their normal rates of activity." It goes on to say that cardiologists at the Oregon Health Sciences University did careful thallium scan testing of D-ribose, which seemed to indicate that it "...was 'waking up' viable areas of heart muscle and helping improve identification of viable ischemic heart muscle."

I was encouraged by the idea that what I'd always thought of as "dead tissue" was really just "hibernating", waiting for the right energy source to bring it back to life so it could repair itself and function again. I didn't know if it could really work that way, having always heard the long-held belief that heart muscle does not regenerate, and that you essentially die with the same heart cells with which you were born.

Something made me decide to check it out.

I was completely unprepared for what I discovered. I had to read it several times before I could even begin to let it sink in.

There it was, on the New York Times website, an article by Nicholas Wade on April 2, 2009, stating that Swedish scientists have proven beyond all doubt that heart muscles do, indeed, regenerate. It's not quick, and their best guess is that only about half of the heart muscle cells do it over the course of an average lifetime, but that's a damn sight better than none, especially with a heart as badly damaged as mine. Over and over again, I stared at the words. I did not believe what I was seeing. I thought it was a prank. I had to check various other websites. I needed to substantiate this story about the team of researchers led by Dr Jonas Frisen at the Karolinska Institute in Stockholm.

When I did, I took off my glasses and laid them on my desk. Then I broke down and cried.

Chapter Twelve

So. It was true. It had been true all along. Heart muscle cells do regencrate, albeit slowly. I could not believe my eyes. For the first time in many years, I had real hope that some of the damage to my heart might actually be healed one day. In fact, combined with other pieces of this self-healing puzzle that will be discussed in later chapters, I had more than enough reason to believe that I could repair every bit of the damage.

I was especially intrigued by results of tests that were done at the High Desert Heart Institute in Victorville, California. Dr Siva Arunasalam, founder and attending cardiologist at the institute has a most impressive educational and employment background, including completing his cardiology training at Cedars-Sinai Medical Center in Los Angeles. Dr Arunasalam conducted an exhaustive study of ProArgi-9+ on 33 extremely ill congestive heart failure patients for whom nothing else could be done. The results were staggering. After just 90 days, these were some of the findings:

* an 18% increase in HDL (good cholesterol)

* a 40% decrease in triglycerides (fatty acids)
* an 8% reduction in blood sugars
* 25% decrease in inflammation in the arteries
* a decrease in platelets (reducing the risk of clotting)
* a 16% increase in peripheral blood flow to the feet
* dramatic decreases in blood pressure.

Dr Arunasalam is quoted as saying "I expected a marginal improvement in the symptoms...what we ended up seeing was remarkable, positive, remodeling of the heart, positive pulmonary artery changes, pulmonary vascular changes..."

People who take this product over a period of months and years report ongoing improvement with the passage of time.

Interestingly, despite the fact that there is no magnesium in the product, there was a 35% increase in magnesium levels, which is extremely important in improving heart health. It would appear that ProArgi-9+ allows the body to better absorb and/or retain this vital mineral, which is the second most abundant element found in human cells and is responsible for hundreds of functions, such as assisting in the production of energy.

Magnesium is partially responsible for DNA repair and the healthy reproduction of cells. When magnesium levels drop, there is an increased chance of cell mutations that can cause critical illness. Magnesium is also extremely important in balancing minerals that affect nerve impulses, muscle contraction and heart rhythms.

After thoroughly researching this product and its various components, I can only say that I felt truly blessed to have found my way to this information and I was happy to begin taking four scoops of this stuff every day. If it was getting people off transplant lists and dramatically improving their health, then it was bound to be a major contributor in my journey toward healing.

But of course, it is not the only contributor. I would still have to get to grips with the basics and that meant addressing one of my biggest daily problems. If you're like most people, it's one of yours, too.

Do you push yourself to keep going, keep working, keep whatevering when you're hungry? Do you skip meals, or rush out the door grabbing something you can shove in your pocket or purse and eat on the way to wherever it is you're going? I've certainly been guilty of this — especially when I've been working on a book. But after what I learned whilst working on this one, I'm not abusing this "Lamborghini in training" any more.

The petrol tank of a car should be kept at least 1/4 full. Less than that, and there may be dirt in the bottom that gets sucked up into the fuel line, which can cause clogging and other problems. Also, the petrol acts as a coolant for the pump, which can fail due to overheating if the tank doesn't have enough fuel in it.

We don't run too well, either, without an adequate source of energy. When we're hungry due to a drop in blood sugar, energy levels drop, leaving us feeling exhausted. We may also experience headaches, lightheadedness, or have trouble concentrating. Such symptoms as these are the only way the body can rebel and remind us that the fuel light is on! It's not good to function this way at all, much less as a regular part of life.

As well as having the proper fuel for its engine type, a car needs to have its various fluid levels maintained, such as oil, transmission fluid, brake fluid and so on. For example, if an engine loses all of its oil for one reason or another, it will seize and be completely destroyed.

Without adequate hydration, the human body suffers, too, and very quickly. We can live for long periods without food if necessary, but we cannot last long without fluids. Obviously, water is extremely important to our health, as it is what makes up 70% of the human body. We begin experiencing symptoms of dehydration when we've lost just 1%-2% of our normal water content. Aside from becoming thirsty, with this seemingly minimal loss of fluid we may also notice fatigue, headaches, dry skin, a loss of appetite, dizziness, confusion, and a change in moods.

With just 5% water loss, there may be overwhelming sleepiness, fainting and seizures. Heart function and respiration are affected in an effort to compensate for the decrease in plasma volume and blood pressure. A loss of more than 15% of our normal water content is usually fatal.

Car parts wear out, their belts break, all sorts of things need to be checked, cleaned, changed or replaced on a regular basis. You are likely to get the most mileage possible from your vehicle with the fewest serious problems if you care for it properly and give it regular maintenance checks.

Likewise, we need to be thinking about the prevention of problems in our bodies by having regular dental visits, blood tests, a checkup now and then to be sure we can nip any potential problems in the bud. But many people keep putting off these kinds of appointments, which only makes things worse as time goes on.

As if this isn't bad enough, we don't stop there. Oh, no, we take a few huge leaps into a very dangerous place, a place that has become "the norm" for far too many people.

With our fast-paced lives, we have an overabundance of "stress hormones" due to too much work and not enough play, and not nearly enough rest. Our busy lives often lead to chronic sleep-deprivation. Too much stress combined with not enough sleep creates a very dangerous combination, and no doubt you and almost everyone you know fits into that category — or at least, will have done for a good portion of the time.

We know we feel miserable when we haven't had enough sleep or when we feel very stressed and pressured. We don't function well physically, running out of energy quickly. We may be more emotional than usual — with irritability, anger, weepiness etc. Mentally, we may struggle with concentration and memory.

Chronic stress and/or sleep loss put the body into stress-response mode on an ongoing basis, thereby creating all sorts of health problems, including weight gain and its associated increased risk factors. To make matters worse, in a stress response state, the body sleeps less, so you get a chicken-and-egg situation. Less sleep equals more stress; more stress equals less sleep. One whole night without sleep produces the same effects as a legally intoxicating blood-alcohol level. We're definitely not functioning at our best in those circumstances.

On a very simple level, when we don't have enough rest, our bodies don't have enough time or energy to take care of the most basic maintenance jobs, such as repairing damaged muscle cells after a workout.

On a more worrisome level, people who do not get enough sleep regularly are at a greater than usual risk for high blood pressure and diabetes. Both of these conditions are potentially threatening for the brain, and of course carry with them the risk of all sorts of problems. Even fields must be left to lie fallow sometimes in order to renew, restore, replenish and be able to produce good crops again.

When the body perceives a threat, its stress-response system kicks in, preparing it for fight or flight. The hypothalamus is a tiny region at the base of the brain, and through a combination of various hormonal and nerve signals, causes the adrenal glands to release hormones, such as adrenaline and cortisol. Once the threat has passed, levels of these hormones return to normal.

However, when you perceive your life as stressful on an ongoing basis, these hormones are continuously being released into your body. Adrenaline increases heart rate and blood pressure, and it also boosts supplies of energy. Cortisol increases the level of glucose in the bloodstream, and its use by the brain. It is part of the system that controls mood and fear. It also diminishes unnecessary or detrimental functions in fight or flight scenarios, such as altering the immune system, suppressing the digestive and reproductive systems, and growth processes.

Imagine how long-term exposure to these hormones could damage your body and many of its processes. It increases your risk of several problems, such as heart disease, depression, obesity, sleep problems, digestive troubles and more.

Just like a car needs to be used frequently to keep it in good working order, daily aerobic physical activity is essential to help burn off these excess stress hormones so they do not attack the body that they are designed to protect. Diet, nutritional supplements (especially antioxidants) as mentioned earlier, and other factors yet to be discussed can work together to reduce the negative effects of stress but our bodies are meant to move and there's no getting around it. Your blood type determines the kind of exercise that is best for you, especially as it relates to reducing stress.

Moreover, we know that regular exercise helps keep joints and muscles in good working order, which reduces the risk of injury. I could never understand that until I was very much out of shape, and managed to hurt myself twisting ever so slightly the wrong way, or lifting something that wasn't even all that heavy. My poor body hadn't a clue what to do with the littlest movement. And using muscles? Did I even *have* any??!

Throughout my life since childhood, I've often heard the old saying "use it or lose it" and I never really appreciated what that meant, until times like those. I had become an adult who detested anything that looked too much like "exercise." I hate sports and even more than that, I hate going to a gym. I've always loved walking, dancing and other physical activity that was enjoyable, but to be honest, I could just as easily enjoy a good, brisk sit...

After all these years, I understand "use it or lose it" now. At one time, I was a young girl who was flexible and quite bendy, doing gymnastics, yoga, and twisting herself into a pretzel. But somewhere along the way, I had become an adult who could no longer touch her toes without a major knee-bending cheat. Muscles stretching? Joints moving easily? Hah! Not a chance. Mobility and flexibility can be regained...with a lot of work (and a fair bit of pain, I should think) but it is so much easier to use them and keep them in the first place!

Generally, in our society, people are far more likely to take better care of their cars than themselves. They listen to weird little noises in their cars; they pay attention when something doesn't sound right or doesn't feel right. But they ignore messages from their own bodies when it is often screaming for food, rest, a 'time out', or they're giving them pain or other symptoms that are trying to say there's a problem.

There's something really wrong with that picture. I reckon it's because there's a more immediate cause and effect situation when something goes wrong with our vehicles, and we rely on them so heavily to get us around. Car runs out of petrol. Car stops. We know we can't coax it into continuing without petrol just a little longer, five more minutes, two more miles please. It has stopped, that's it, and we are forced to give it what it needs.

But then Human runs out of energy. Human ignores its own warning light. Ignores gauge falling below "E". Human digs deeper, runs on fumes and keeps going till it feels like hell or something Really Big goes wrong.

Transmission in car quits. Gotta get that fixed right now or that car ain't goin' nowhere. But Human? Human gets the flu. Feels absolutely miserable. Aching, feverish, lethargic, hacking its lungs out. But every morning, Human takes some cold or flu meds or Tylenol, stuffs itself into its clothes and takes itself, its sore throat, its congestion, sneezing, and all those hearty little germs to work, where it can share them with everyone else.

And then it gripes because it gets sicker. Or it takes way too long to recover. Or (c) both of the above. It might even feel like its body has failed it by becoming ill, and is making things worse by taking its sweet time to get well. Yes, Humans are indeed that arrogant.

Many people go without enough sleep, a proper diet, or enough water on a regular basis. Sadly, it is typical in the West. We get away with living a less-than-healthy lifestyle as long as possible, accepting aches and pains, fatigue, poor sleep and stress-related symptoms as normal parts of aging and/or life in general.

Most of us do not ever stop to consider exactly what is going on in our bodies as we move through our lives. We shovel in whatever food strikes our fancy, dash out the door to work, carry on with our jobs, responsibilities, family life. If we're lucky, we allow a little down time, too, before falling into bed exhausted at night, only do it all again the next day.

We don't usually stop to consider the countless processes that are going on every moment that we're breathing, whether we're thinking about them or not. And we are certainly not thinking about what is required in order for those processes to happen. Yet we expect that somehow, despite the way we neglect, or in fact abuse ourselves, our bodies will perform perfectly. We demand strength and endurance. And we can become quite annoyed when it doesn't work out like that. Too often, we treat our bodies with disrespect, and have the audacity to turn on ourselves and feel betrayed by our bodies when we run into problems with our health.

Do you recognise yourself anywhere in here so far? Most certainly, I do.

For a moment, stop and think about your body. Think about its various parts, both internal and external. Every one of those parts is made up of cells. There are trillions of them in your whole body. Do you ever consider what they're doing whilst you're going about your business? Those cells are busy transporting oxygen, carbon dioxide, proteins and more. They are busy creating energy and using it to keep you alive, breathing, moving. They are busy cleaning house, best they can, against the pollutants, drugs, and other toxic rubbish that you are ingesting, inhaling, or that is created by your body as waste, whilst it's busy working for you every moment of your life.

Your brain cells are constantly sending messages to every other cell in your body and they respond in kind, with an astonishing and brilliant rapid-fire communication system. There are muscle cells helping you move — voluntary ones like in your arms and legs, involuntary ones like in your stomach and intestinal tract.

There are blood cells, racing through every part of your body, dispersing oxygen to every cell and collecting carbon dioxide for you to exhale. Your heart cells are beating, one electrical impulse after another in unison to keep you alive. And they've been doing it non-stop, day and night, without a break since you were just a tiny embryo.

That cells just seem to know what to do is truly a marvel. For example, in the small intestine, there are several different types of epithelial cells, some of which absorb nutrients, some secrete digestive enzymes, while still others secrete a protective mucous. Virtually all substances that enter or leave the body must cross at least one epithelial layer. Each cell must always transport a substance in only one of two directions: either from blood vessels outside to the hollow interior (**lumen**) inside, or from the lumen out to the blood vessels. Therefore, the cells must have a "sense of direction." They have to "know" which is the blood side and which is the lumen side.

I could write whole chapters on cell function, on how they transport nutrients, chemicals, lipids, water and more, into and out of themselves and between one another. I could write about their life cycles, how the various types of cells reproduce, when, and why. I could write about all their tiny little parts, called organelles, or their 'bones and muscles' called cytoskeletons, which give them their shapes.

They are astonishing; there is so much to say about them, and about their magnificent abilities, but it is not necessary for the purposes of this book. It is enough to know that they are incredibly complex, and to remember that without them, we would not exist.

We must also be mindful that they require adequate rest, nourishment and fluid to fulfill their many tasks, and as you will see in later chapters, many other aspects of our lives influence what happens in the lives of our cells. Without them, we die. If we give them the respect and care that they deserve, they will allow us to accomplish many things throughout our lives.

How do cells know what to do? Their lives and jobs are very complex. How do they work? For example, how are they nourished? How do they dispose of waste? How do they recognise invaders or anything else that is harmful and requires clean-up and disposal?

Or did you ever wonder just how it is that if you cut your leg, cells elsewhere in your body know about it? And how do they know they're meant to race to that area and do something to fix it?

Damaged cells in the area of the cut send out a chemical "alarm", which is picked up by receptors on white blood cells that circulate through the body like police monitoring the blood for any intruders. Instantly, white cells rush to the site.

No road map, no mobiles, no sat-nav, yet somehow they just know where to go —and they know what to do when they get there. Microbes (germs) that entered the body via the cut will be consumed by the white cells. Other cells will begin sealing the hole, repairing the damage and creating new skin cells. It seems simple enough on the surface, but if you think about it for a moment, it is truly astonishing. It's as though cells can think...but how can that be?

Chapter Thirteen

B ruce Lipton, Ph.D. conducted research on cloned endothelial cells, the cells that line blood vessels. He discovered that they monitor their environment very closely, and change their behaviour based on the information they gather. When nutrients were introduced into their environment, the cells gravitated toward them. But when a toxic environment was created, the cells retreated, moving away from the dangerous substances.

In an effort to understand what was controlling these shifts in behaviour, Lipton studied the membrane perception switches. There are two types of switches: H1 and H2, both of which contain a protein that responds to histamine, a molecular alarm bell, of sorts, in the body. H1 histamine receptors produce a protective response, whilst H2 histamine receptors produce a growth response.

Further, Lipton studied adrenalin, which is a "system-wide" emergency response signal sent out under the orders of the central nervous system (CNS). He discovered that it, too, has two different receptors: one that produces a protection response when adrenalin is detected, and another that produces a growth response.

What makes this particularly interesting is that when both histamine and adrenalin were introduced to the cell cultures simultaneously, "system-wide" adrenalin signals overrode the more local histamine signals. It would appear that our bodies have a built-in "intelligence" that forces cells to follow instructions sent out by the CNS, whatever messages they are receiving locally.

Therefore, although local cells will react to what is going on in their immediate environment, they will change their behaviour according to orders received by the CNS.

Lipton has established that both growth and protection behaviours are essential for our survival (and indeed, for the survival of other organisms as well) but cells cannot respond to both signals at once. It would be likened to trying to go forward and backward at the same time; it is physically impossible.

For example, when the fight or flight response is required, growth behaviours are restricted, as all energy reserves are directed to do what is necessary for protection (i.e. fighting or fleeing).

The problem with this is that although the growth process requires an expenditure of energy, it is also necessary to produce energy. Therefore, when we are in protection mode for an extended period of time, it has a profoundly negative impact on our ability to create life-sustaining energy. Certainly, we are able to survive short periods of stress and recover fully once the stressors are removed and we are back in growth mode again.

However, chronic stress means ongoing suppression of the growth response, which severely compromises health and vitality. Clearly, we are designed to thrive in positive, nurturing environments that are free of stressful, negative conditions.

Interestingly, this is not at all the only situation in which we see evidence of this. Others will be discussed in later chapters.

There is another aspect to the life cycle of a cell that must be addressed because it is also essential to keeping us well, and sometimes contributes to making us ill. I'm talking about cell death. What causes cells to die? How can this keep us well? More importantly, how can this make us ill?

Liberty Forrest

In adults, for various reasons, approximately 50 to 70 billion cells die every day. One cause is cell necrosis, which occurs when a cell is damaged due to trauma, as in an injury, and its contents spill out into the surrounding area.

Programmed cell death (apoptosis), on the other hand, is a very specifically organised series of steps that lead to the deaths of certain cells that for one reason or another must die. At times, they must shut down and stop production, a process that is necessary for the proper development and maintenance of all multi-cellular organisms. However, despite the body's best-laid plans, sometimes things go awry, and flaws in the apoptotic process can lead to disease or disorders.

Phagocytic molecules, such as phosphatidylserine, appear on the surfaces of dying cells, marking them for phagocytosis, a process by which cells such as macrophages recognise the markers and begin the process of engulfing - and thereby removing - the dying cells.

The whole process requires a range of cell signals, which originate either extracellularly or intracellularly. Extracellular signals include the effects of growth factors, hormones, toxins or oxidative damage. Intracellular apoptotic signals occur in response to some form of stress, such as radiation, nutrient deprivation, heat or a lack of oxygen.

As several steps are required to take a cell from initiating apoptosis to its actual death, there are various points at which the process can be halted. In some cases, it is because the cell no longer needs to die. In others, there is a fault and a cell that should die continues to live.

This causes a number of problems, including many cancers, as well as autoimmune and inflammatory diseases. Previous studies in these fields showed that there was an increase in the proliferation of cells, which was believed to be the cause of these diseases. However, with more recent research into apoptosis, now we know that it is also due to a decrease in the number of cells that should have died, which allows them to create all manner of problems.

Just as inhibiting apoptosis can create diseases and disorders, so the opposite is also true. When too many cells have become programmed to die, we see degenerative diseases that affect numerous systems in the body, from blood to bone to soft tissue. Wasting diseases, such as ALS, Huntington's disease and even some of the damage that occurs after a stroke are just a few examples of diseases in which apoptosis has occurred too quickly for the body to compensate by producing the necessary number of healthy cells to restore balance. In AIDS, the disease progresses mainly as a result of an excessive depletion of T-helper cells and the bone marrow cannot replace them at an equally high rate to keep the patient well.

When you consider how your body knew to create itself, that each cell knows what it needs to do, when to reproduce, and even when it is time to die - or even trickier, that it knows when to stop the process of dying if it is no longer required — it is impossible to dispute the idea of cell intelligence.

You started out as two cells that merged as one, which began to divide, as did all the others after it. Have you ever thought about the fact that those cells looked like an unidentifiable blob for a week or two, with each cell looking the same as all the others? But then gradually, that blob began to change shape. And the cells became different from one another.

How did they know to do that? They were all the same, copies made again and again as they divided, but suddenly, some of them began to change. Just a few weeks in, you had a brain with its main sections identifiable, and you had a tube-shaped heart.

By four weeks, that heart was beating. You had a central nervous system, a liver, a neck and limb buds. By six weeks, you had a face, a mouth, feet, tips of toes. You had eyes, ears and moving hands. You still looked rather blob-like, but gradually, you were beginning to look sort of human.

At seven weeks, tiny bones such as in your hands, wrists and spine could have been seen. You had knees. You had eyelids and irises. You had a little nose. You were only about half an inch long. But you had all of these parts. And more.

By nine weeks, you looked decidedly human at just one and a half inches long. Over the following weeks and months, of course you continued to develop, with all of your various parts maturing until eventually, your body could function outside of your mother's womb.

Most of us take all of this for granted. Most of us don't stop to ponder how it happens that each of us begins as one cell that miraculously begins dividing into all of these separate and amazing, highly complex and interdependent working parts. What is it that makes certain newly created cells "know" that they are destined to become liver cells or kidney cells or blood vessels?

And then, how does each liver cell know which part of the liver it is meant to be? A part of the hepatic vein? Perhaps a bit of the membrane that separates the right and left lobes? Or one of the ligaments that connects it to the diaphragm? Or maybe that cell decides to become part of the bile ducts, which comprise one third of the liver.

And as if it isn't enough that all of your cells know precisely which kinds of cells they should become, they also know just how to work. Whatever you're doing, awake or asleep, every single cell is busy with its particular tasks, automatically carrying out its own significant contribution to the growth, repair, maintenance or function of your body. In the case of the liver, the organ as a whole carries out over 500 functions in the body. Can you imagine what a miracle it is that each of those cells knows just which part of what job it is intended to do? And then does it?

We say it's just "Mother Nature." We are so used to just getting on with our lives and not thinking about the millions of miracles that are being performed in our bodies by trillions of cells at any given moment that we do not consider the magnitude of these processes. Every cell is intelligent. Every one of them knows exactly what to be, what to do and how to heal. But to us, it's just DNA creating and replicating, something we've heard about so often and for such a long time, we think it's no big deal. Most of us never even consider for one moment exactly what is involved.

But it's time we did consider it. We must sit up and take notice of the inherent power and the potential, both positive and negative, which are available to us in every single cell of our bodies. After decades of research around the globe, it has become abundantly clear that we are dealing with cell intelligence, an innate and intelligent creative power that goes beyond the physical, the material. This is but one piece of a fascinating puzzle, whose completed picture will prove to you beyond the shadow of a doubt that we are capable of healing any disease or disorder ourselves.

But how?

On one hand, I'm telling you that our cells have all this creative intelligence and that in every moment of our lives, they're busy getting on with what they're meant to be doing. But on the other hand, I'm telling you that we have the ability to heal ourselves. So how has that got anything to do with us? Just exactly how can we heal ourselves if our cells are calling all the shots?

Chapter Fourteen

I f we're going to understand how we can heal ourselves, first, we must accept the creative intelligence of our cells, our bodies. It is true that every cell knows how to grow, and how to repair itself and so on. As we're already aware, most of our bodies' functions are taking place without our notice, whether we're awake, asleep or paying them any attention at all. But I have not suggested for one moment that our cells are calling all the shots.

Well, then, just what is this creative intelligence? Is it some incredible, magical feat of nature or of the universe? Is it what some people would call God?

To be honest, we don't know. And there's not much point in wondering about what it is or how it came to be, because even if we knew the answer to either of those questions, human nature would make us wonder what created the force that created cell intelligence. And then we would want to know what created the force, and then what created *that* one, and so on. For some things, there are simply no answers for our human brains.

It does not really matter what this creative intelligence is, or how it came to be. We can give it many names and speculate about possible explanations, but the only bit that is of any real importance for our purposes here is the fact that we know it exists. Clearly, there is a powerful force at work, creating our bodies and all of our organs, and causing our hearts to beat and our brains to function. That creative force is responsible for all of us being here, alive, breathing, and growing.

While we're doing all of that living and breathing and growing, the human body is like a rainfall. You look out the window and see a whole lot of raindrops falling, splattering, bouncing.

A year later, you look out the window at another rainfall. You think "So what? Another rainfall, just like every other one." As you've seen so many times before, raindrops are falling, bouncing off the pavement, pecking at small puddles, like the beaks of invisible chickens.

But you have not seen ***this*** rainfall before. These are not the same raindrops as the ones you saw last year. Or the ones you saw just a moment ago, or will five minutes from now. Each one of those raindrops is different from all the others that have existed. In every moment that you're looking out that window, you're seeing millions and millions of new raindrops. The view is not really the same after all; it only appears to be.

There are approximately 200 different types of cells in the many trillions that make up your body. Most types of cells die, only to be replaced. We look essentially the same from one day to the next, but in every moment, cells are dying, whilst new ones are being created. Some cells, such as certain blood cells, live for just a few hours, whilst others, like nerve cells, last your whole lifetime, and do not regenerate. Some muscle cells live for just a few days.

Others remain unchanged for a person's whole life. Skin cells live for only one month. White blood cells for two days; red ones for four months. Brain cells for 60 years or more. Surface stomach cells are renewed every five minutes. One year from now, 98% of the atoms in your body right now will have been replaced.

Outwardly, you'll look about the same as you do now. But you'll be like those raindrops, constantly changing in every moment. Even cancer cells constantly die and are replaced, so that if you had a tumour now, in a year it would not be the same cancer, the same tumour.

In cancer, a distorted cell "blueprint", or memory, has been created, and as each cell dies, new ones are created based on that blueprint. It's a bit like setting a photocopier to produce 100 copies of a document. You walk away and return later, only to discover that partway through the process, there was a fault. The blank sheets were not properly lined up in the tray, so they've come out with the printing all askew on the page.

Or for some reason the copies are blurred and illegible. But the copier doesn't know this. It keeps producing copy and after copy, each one being printed according to the instructions it was given, but they no longer look anything like the original.

In cancer, somewhere along the way, cells have run amok in their reproduction process, and the new cells continue to be created based on the instructions they are given.

The good news is that this means we can fix the copier and eliminate further defective ones. But I'm getting ahead of myself.

We lose an average of 18 million neurons (nerve cells) a year after age 30. As they are responsible for brain function, after that time you would expect a gradual increase in symptoms of "old age" such as impaired memory, or an inability to reason. But this has turned not to be the case. Interestingly, early research was always done on the elderly who were ill and in hospital. Their memories were poor; many showed symptoms of senility. But later studies of healthy elderly people show no significant memory impairment. It was determined that new information is not retained as well as in younger people, but long-term memory actually improves.

Further, when memory exercises were practiced in tests on 70-year-olds for just a few minutes on a daily basis, their results almost equalled those of the 20-year-olds who were at their peak of mental performance.

How is this possible if they were losing millions of neurons every year since they were 30?

It is because the body, in all its creative wisdom, compensates for this loss by growing new dendrites, thin tree-like "arms" that branch out from nerve cells, allowing them to continue communicating. There may be only a few dendrites on a cell, or more than one thousand, depending on how many are required for nerve cells to send signals to one another as their numbers gradually decrease. The greater the number of dendrites we have, the more connected our nerve cells are, which keeps our brains functioning.

Interestingly, as dendrites increase in number, allowing more connectedness between nerve cells than ever before, our thoughts begin to connect experience and learning, bringing a deeper understanding of our lives, ourselves, and each other. And what else is this besides wisdom?

In fact, perhaps the decrease in neurons and the increase in dendrites is not a compensatory measure after all. Perhaps it is a necessary step in the process of gaining wisdom.

How fascinating it is, then, to consider that our brain cells seem to "know" when to stop working so hard to retain new information, and instead, they change how they function, and begin to communicate in a way that may suggest they are using old information in a newer and more meaningful way, bringing a richness to our lives that only comes with wisdom.

This is the intelligence of our cells — our bodies — at its very best.

If such an intelligent power can create an entire human being with all of its intricate functions, changing them according to our needs, moment by moment throughout our lives, then it would seem that repairing a few damaged or malfunctioning parts ought to be fairly simple. And if this intelligent force is responsible for creating every cell in our bodies, it is also responsible for creating cells that become tumours.

Likewise, if it is responsible for the creation of chemicals that flow through our bodies, communicating from one organ or system to another, it is also responsible for creating imbalances in these chemicals, and thereby causing disease or disorders.

As mentioned in Chapter 3, chemical messengers, such as neurotransmitters and neuropeptides, are "communicator molecules", which allow the neurons in the brain to communicate with the rest of the body. They are found in abundance in the amygdala and the hypothalamus, areas of the brain that govern our emotions.

In the 1980s, the National Institute of Mental Health discovered that there are receptors for these neurotransmitters outside the brain. For example, many were found on monocytes, cells that are part of the immune system. These cells circulate in the bloodstream, relaying messages freely throughout the body, and not just from one neuron to the next along the fixed path of the CNS, as was previous thought. But rather, they have free access to every other cell in the body and therefore, as they are receptors for neurotransmitters, they carry the messages of our emotions.

These chemicals carry every feeling, every wish, every hope, every fear from the brain where they were created, to every single cell in the body. You do not merely store them in your consciousness. Those memories, thoughts and feelings are stored in every single part of your body.

Take a moment to think about an emotional memory — perhaps a particularly beautiful one, or a tragic one, or a traumatic one. If you pay attention to what's going on physically as a result of those thoughts, you will notice that your entire body is affected. One need only watch someone who's excited and happy, and you can see body language reflecting this. There's a big smile on her face; she's beaming. There's a spring in her step, or perhaps she is giggling and bouncing up and down like a little kid, unable to remain still.

Now consider the body language of someone who is depressed. His head hangs. His shoulders droop. He may have a furrowed brow, and the corners of his mouth are turned down. He walks slowly, seems to have no energy. He may have terrible headaches, stomach pain, or pain in his joints and elsewhere. He may be spending count-less miserable hours in bed in a darkened room.

Have you ever experienced overwhelming anxiety, as you antici-pate something scary? Perhaps a crucial exam, or "meeting his/her parents"? Do you know that awful tight knot in the pit of your stom-ach? The sweaty palms? Dry mouth? Racing heart?

Your thoughts have no physical substance; they can't be seen, touched or photographed. They're intangible. Yet they are absolutely and profoundly linked to your physical body. We have scientific evidence that our infinite creative intelligence has a direct and prov-able effect on the physical body. Every thought you have is coded into a chemical message, which is then relayed via neurotransmitters to every cell in the body.

The short version: Your thoughts will manifest in your physical body.

How do we know this? After all, as stated above, a thought has no substance. It cannot be touched. But it can be "seen" in the form of ink on a graph, an electromagnetic wave detectable on an electroen-cephalogram (EEG). And although it is not a tangible thing, a neuro-transmitter is. Its job is to create matter where there was none. Neurotransmitters must be as flexible and changeable as the thoughts that create them.

In order to respond to a potentially infinite number of these messages, DNA continuously creates receptors that reach up like long fingers to the surfaces of cells. Each receptor is like an eye, looking out from the cell for one specific message. Therefore, recep-tors are not fixed; sometimes cells have none at all, while at other times they are loaded with them, depending upon how many messages the cell needs to "see."

We know that people with depression have abnormally high levels of a neurotransmitter called imipramine in their brains. Not only are there imipramine receptors on their brain cells, but on skin cells, as well. Similarly, anxious people have very high levels of epinephrine and norepinephrine in their brains, as well as abnormal concentrations of both of these chemicals in their blood platelets.

Therefore, we can assume from this, and similar findings in other research, that the whole body "feels" the thoughts we think. And we know that what we think creates how we feel. I will go into this in much more detail in later chapters. But it does explain — at least in part — why I noticed an immediate improvement in my ailments by "speaking to them" when I began going for walks at the start of this self-healing project.

Not only do our thoughts and feelings affect the living cells we have at any given moment, new cells are being created using the current "blueprint", a plan generated by your consciousness. That plan is the result of your thoughts, making you the architect of your cells, their memories, their programming, their behaviour — and your health.

Thoughts can be habitual, and as with any habit, it can take time to change them. It's like moving house. You take all of your belongings to a new environment, and absentmindedly, you keep turning left instead of right to get to the kitchen, forgetting that it's on the other side of the hallway now. Or reaching into the cupboard next to the sink for a glass, only to discover that they're in a new place in this house. But with new information, it doesn't take long for us to adapt and make changes to our behaviour.

When we change our thoughts, we change the chemical messages that the brain is sending. Therefore, our cells are given new information, a new "blueprint", and they will reproduce according to those instructions.

But before we can learn how to do that, we must explore the labyrinths of one of the most mysterious and powerful creations in the known universe, as our adventure takes us deep into the heart of a very secret, and very hidden place. A place no one has ever seen.

And no one ever will.

Chapter Fifteen

J ust where is this secret place? How do we know it exists if no one has ever seen it? And what has it got to do with self-healing?

This secret place is buried deep within you. Every experience you've ever had is safely tucked away, some of it so safely, in fact, that you haven't seen it or thought about it in many years. And much of it may never see daylight again.

This secret place is your subconscious mind. And it has everything to do with the state of your health — and with self-healing.

How is that possible, you ask? If you don't even know what's in there, how can you possibly have any control over it? And how on earth can it be responsible for your health?

Bear with me, please. This is an enormous topic, but we'll get through it one step at a time.

The subconscious is the storehouse for all of our memories. Every word that has ever been spoken to us, or by us, every experience we've ever had — even experiences we had in the womb and as babies or small children. If we have consciousness, we have also got awareness. We may not always understand what is happening around us, or to us, but we are still aware. It's like watching a foreign film without subtitles.

For example, if we are subjected to anger and violence as babies or toddlers, we do not have words to put on what we saw, or on how we felt. At that stage of life, if we're listening to arguments and fighting, we don't understand the words being spoken or shouted. But we can feel every bit of the fear. Our eyes see intimidating gestures, threatening or violent acts and we understand without needing it explained.

Even without words, we can still be traumatised by many experiences, simply because we have witnessed them. And these become our memories. Every single moment of our lives has been locked away in the darkest recesses of our minds, whether our conscious minds remember them or not.

As a certified hypnotist, I have had occasion to study the subconscious and to work with it in many clients since the mid-90s. I've certainly seen evidence of the well-established fact that the subconscious mind is running the show. We know it is responsible for our emotional responses, and that they dictate our actions. Awake or asleep, the subconscious is constantly reacting to our everyday lives, to the events that occur and the circumstances in which we live.

It's a sort of auto-pilot, like the operating system in a computer, quietly running (often amok) in the background much of the time. It is the filter through which we view every thought we think, every experience we have, every choice we make.

For example, if a child has been viciously attacked by a dog, it is quite likely that such an incident will leave a lasting impression, causing the child — and later, the adult — to become terrified by every other dog he sees again. In a heartbeat, those fears will rise to the surface, flooding the conscious mind with memories of the attack, which trigger a sense of panic and a certainty that another attack is imminent.

If the subconscious mind is so powerful, and it is operating 24/7, how on earth can we tame this unruly beast? Surely, it must be impossible. After all, it has all the control. Hasn't it?

I suppose it might seem that way. On the one hand, I'm telling you that the subconscious functions with a will of its own, throwing out one automatic response after another, and we don't seem to have any control over it, whatsoever. And on the other hand, I'm telling you that it is at the heart of our ability to heal ourselves. If that's the case, just how is it supposed to work if we cannot control it?

I did not say we cannot control it. It's just that most of the time, we *do not* control it — because we don't know that we can, or we don't know how to do it. The subconscious is merely reacting to the information that it has been fed by the conscious mind throughout our lives. Because most of us don't understand how this works, we are not aware that the subconscious can be programmed — or perhaps reprogrammed — to do what we want it to do.

Your conscious mind gathers information from your external world. Everything that happens around you, or to you, every word that you hear, every incident you witness, every wonderful or frightening experience that you have, all of it is collected by the conscious mind, which then uses logic and reason to draw conclusions about you and the world around you. These conclusions are beliefs that the conscious mind deposits into the "bank" of your subconscious, where they remain unless and until they are replaced with new ones.

For example, if a child is raised in a loving and nurturing environment, he'll believe the world is safe and he'll react accordingly. He will be a secure and happy child. He will trust easily.

Imagine, then, what would happen in the face of a terrible tragedy. What if someone broke into the child's home and murdered one or both parents in front of him? Can you imagine how this would change his beliefs about the world? He would no longer be a secure and happy child. He might become frightened of strangers. Even in his own home, he would be terrified of someone breaking in. His conscious mind would have witnessed this terrible event and concluded that the world is a frightening violent place, and he would believe that he's not even safe in his own home.

With such beliefs as those locked away in the subconscious, you can imagine how they would affect this child's choices and feelings — right the way through to adulthood. What might he be like as a grown man? He might become violent himself, as a way of getting round being vulnerable, or he may be lashing out because of long-buried rage.

On the other hand, he may be terrified of violence and keep himself locked up in his home as much as possible, hoping he is safe behind barred windows and several deadbolts on the doors. He would probably have enormous trust issues, which would make it difficult for him to have relationships. Not simply because of a traumatic incident that he witnessed, but because of what he came to believe about the world and everyone else in it as a result of that incident.

With proper therapy, a new perspective and the right kind of support, he may become a relatively "normal" adult who will of course always remember what happened, but will not allow it to adversely affect his choices or his life.

Sometimes we don't understand our responses to particular situations. Often, they are due to long-buried incidents from the past. Obviously, they left an impression at the time, and even though the conscious mind does not recall those incidents, the subconscious does, as it records absolutely everything. Or we may have a general understanding of our self-destructive behaviour, knowing that it is the result of years of emotional abuse and criticism.

Every belief you have is hard at work at all times, whether or not you're thinking about them, whether or not you're even aware that they exist. Firmly planted in the subconscious, our beliefs create that operating system that affects every thought we think, every choice we make. Unless we pay attention to them and consciously change our beliefs, we will continue to surround ourselves with people and situations that validate them. We become caught in a chicken-and-egg cycle. Thought creates belief; belief creates thought.

We may feel as though we have no control over these responses, because we cannot go back to the past and undo what was done to us. We think we're stuck with the memories and its harmful effects on our lives.

This is where we are wrong. Of course we cannot go back in time, but we **can** undo the resulting damage that has been caused by a painful past. There are several ways in which this can be done, some of them overlapping in theory, and many of which will be covered in this book.

We begin by looking at beliefs. Not specific ones, of course, but the idea of beliefs in general, and the impact they have on our lives. One of the most important misconceptions about beliefs is that people often think they are the same as facts, when in actuality there is a world of difference between the two. A belief is merely an opinion that is held to be true — an opinion, and nothing more. A fact is provable, consistent and indisputable.

Ask any child about the existence of Father Christmas or the Easter Bunny and he will tell you that they are as real as you are. This is what he has been told is the truth and he believes it, despite never having seen any actual evidence. This is his opinion. But two plus two will always equal four. We can prove this readily enough and we will always get the same result. It is a fact.

As a child, I was told repeatedly that I was stupid. I was told I was ugly, that I would never amount to anything, and frequently my mother said, "I just want to get rid of you!" I was told I did not deserve good things, nice boyfriends. "What would a great guy like *that* see in someone like *you*?!"

I agreed with everything my mother said about me; I had no reason to believe it wasn't the truth. From the moment I was adopted, there was a lot in the way she treated me and spoke to me that validated what she said about me. When she wasn't saying the words, I was thinking them to myself.

All of those thoughts filtered down into my subconscious mind, the womb of emotions and behaviours, the birthplace of every choice I made.

I grew up believing I was worthless, stupid, undeserving of anything good. I had plenty of trouble in relationships, to say the least, and it took many years to unravel everything that went into the countless poor choices I made in my life. For decades, I heard my mother's voice echoing through my head, telling me "You don't deserve...", "You're not good enough...", "You should be ashamed of yourself!"

And after one particularly abusive relationship, she said to me, "Don't you think you and your kids deserved all that abuse? You're pretty hard to take!"

I believed she was wrong about my children and I defended them, telling her they didn't deserve it. But I had no reason to think she was wrong about me so I didn't defend myself. I'd had many years to believe that she was right. After all, she was my mother. She *must* have been right. Mustn't she? Her opinions and treatment of me created the thoughts I had about myself and my life, and ultimately, these became the belief system upon which I had built an extremely turbulent life.

Our beliefs shape our thoughts. Our thoughts shape our choices. And our choices shape our lives. Therefore, what you are thinking about will ultimately create your reality. You will read these words more than once in this book because it is imperative that you understand how important they are.

To demonstrate this, I'd like to introduce you to Albert Ellis, a psychologist, who, in the 1950s, developed what he called Rational Emotive Therapy. It is the foundation for what we now call Cognitive Behavioural Therapy, and was based on what he called the ABC Theory: "A" (an action, or event) leads to "B" (a belief about the event), which leads to "C" (the consequence, or response to the event). He said that usually, we think that "A" leads directly to "C".

Let's say, for example, that your spouse smacks you hard across the face. If you were raised in a loving home in which this sort of thing was unheard of, it's likely that in the same instant, you would become hurt and angry. You might ring the police, pack a bag and leave. But what if you were raised in a home where this sort of behaviour was normal, and your parents hit each other — and you — on a regular basis? If your spouse slapped you, in all likelihood you would just carry on as normal, even if you didn't particularly like what had happened.

In both cases, it appears as though "A" — the slap — leads to "C" — the emotional response. But quick as a wink, jammed in tightly between the two is "B", the belief about the slap.

In the first example, there's a belief that this is just wrong, this is shocking, this is unacceptable, and therefore, you would respond accordingly. But in the second example, there's a belief that this is entirely normal. You'd think this is how married people behave. It is to be expected. You don't have to like it, but it's just the way things are. And so you continue to put up with it.

You can see from this example how quietly, yet powerfully, our beliefs drive our behaviour and choices. We don't even notice them, yet they are always there, creating constant and instantaneous links between the events of our lives and how we respond to them.

There's a chicken-and-egg thing with our thoughts and beliefs, too. Once you have certain beliefs, they are the foundation for your thoughts. And the more you persist with those thoughts, the more you strengthen those beliefs.

Anything that's repeated regularly becomes a habit, whether a thought or an activity. If we have the power to create negative or harmful habits, we have also got the power to create positive ones.

Our feelings are usually directly related to what we're thinking about. If you want to change how you're feeling, you've got to change your thoughts. When we're feeling trapped by a "negative emotion", such as fear or depression, it's as though it has us in a death grip and we have no control over it. But this is often a false belief. It might not happen in a minute or two, and it may not be overnight either. I am well acquainted with depression, for example, and I know that being in a happy circumstance or plastering on a smile does not make it go away. It takes more than that, and that's the point I'm trying to make.

Staying with the example of depression, let's say you're in a deep, dark pit of it. You go to a social event, a party or celebration of some kind. You tell yourself a few times — perhaps even several — that you'll have a good time, that it'll be fun. But these thoughts are immediately wiped out with the negatives. "I still feel really miserable." "I can't fake being happy." "I don't really want to be there." "It'll take so much energy to get through this and try to pretend I'm enjoying it."

And please hear me, I'm not minimising depression or how difficult it is to live with that heaviness and those thoughts. I'm just saying... there is often a component that can at least be improved, if not significantly helped, but it takes time. I've lived it, too; I respect the suffering and how difficult this is. I'm also aware that it can help.

It takes a consistent effort to monitor all those negative thoughts, to push each one away as it comes to you and replace it with a positive idea, an affirmation, a word or two of hope. I know it can be overwhelming to imagine doing this. It's as though you're looking at a 40-foot buffet table, filled with plates and trays full of food, and you feel like you have to eat every bit of that food, right now — and you'll never get there. It can feel like "Why bother? I'll never finish, so I'm not even going to start."

But you must. It's worth a solid attempt. One negative thought at a time, gradually you can change how you feel. We have a lot more control over what goes on in our heads than we might think we do. We're just not used to thinking that way. We *believe* (there's that word again) that thoughts just randomly drift into our heads and we're stuck with them, whatever they are, for better or worse.

But this is not so. It's true that thoughts wander in without an invitation, but we don't have to let them stay and go down the road of entertaining a whole bunch of others just like them. We can show them the door and invite other ones that work *for* us, and not *against* us.

Your perspective is a function of your beliefs and it makes all the difference in the world. You get to choose what it is. It's that "glass half-empty/half-full" thing. You can decide to look at a difficult situation with dread, adopting a gloom and doom attitude, or you can decide to find the positives in it, to see it as a big adventure, a challenge with opportunities for growth. You can choose to accept change and go with the flow of life. Or not.

At this point in numerous discussions with clients, patients, friends and family down the years, many of them have disagreed with me about that. "But I have clinical depression, caused by a chemical imbalance!" Or "Anxiety runs in my family!" Or "Of course I'm going to feel really stressed! Look at the mess my life is in right now!"

Well, perhaps the gene pool makes a person more susceptible to certain emotions. Or perhaps they learned to respond a certain way because that's what was done in the family and they saw that this was how everyone around them lived. And yes, changes in body chemistry go hand-in-hand with anxiety, depression, stress, and all other emotions, both positive and negative. I am not disputing any of this. Actually, it helps to prove an earlier point I made in this book — that the whole body "feels" what we're thinking about. Is it another of those chicken-and-egg situations?

Perhaps. Which one came first is irrelevant, to be honest, but one thing is certain: Once you're in that negative place, if you keep thinking depressing, anxious or stressful thoughts, you will alter your chemistry accordingly. As I explained in an earlier chapter, our thoughts create chemical messengers, and those have a massive impact on making us to feel happy, anxious, depressed etc.

The bottom line is the same: ultimately, whatever state you're in right now, if you are suffering from depression or prolonged grief due to terrible losses, if you are anxious and having panic attacks, if you are stressed so that your blood pressure is through the roof and you're having loads of headaches and feeling burned out, "wired" etc., you can still change how you're feeling if you just change your thoughts. Consistently, one at a time.

Don't think about eating every bit of food on every single tray on that 40-foot buffet table. You need only to begin with one bite of the food on just that one tray, right there, in front of you. Then another bite, and another. When you do this, one thought at a time, gradually you will begin to feel better, and this new way of thinking gathers momentum. The more positive thoughts you have, the easier they come to you.

I can speak from a lifetime of personal experience with this. I've overcome several difficult and seemingly impossible challenges by changing my thoughts. Although it is but one piece of the huge puzzle I'm putting together for you in this book, it's a significant one. As a "stand-alone" bit of help, it can work wonders, but you'll see in later chapters how it can be applied in specific ways that make it far more powerful.

It is said that a journey of a thousand miles begins with one step, although a more accurate translation from the original Chinese quotation by Lao-Tzu, the Father of the Tao, is that it begins beneath one's feet. I remember all too well the torment and fear that were beneath mine at one time. It was before I knew there could be another way, when I thought that's all there would ever be for me.

I saw only that journey of a thousand miles, yet I didn't know that that "one step" even existed for me. And in the moment I realised that I had an addiction, that journey might as well have been to the moon.

Chapter Sixteen

As the most vulnerable member of my family, I took the brunt of the anger, alcoholism and abuse that were part of my everyday existence whilst growing up. Aching to please and always trying to be "the good girl", I kept hoping that maybe one day, I would be "good enough" to deserve the warmth, the affection and the love I needed so desperately. But it was not meant to be.

Instead, my days were filled with anxiety, always waiting for the next insult, the next slap, kick or punch, the next violation. The atmosphere was fairly vibrating with tension, every waking moment - and even whilst I slept. As a tiny child, I had terrifying nightmares and I learned very quickly not to disturb my parents on those all-too-frequent occasions.

By the age of nine, I was waking with violent panic attacks, although it would be many long years before I knew what was happening. I lay alone in my bed, shaking so wildly that I couldn't hold a glass of water, much less drink it. I was utterly terrified, filled with a sense of dread that flooded through my body. With my heart racing, I was certain that I would die. But I didn't dare go to my parents.

I could understand my terrified shaking in the night when I woke to the sounds of my parents fighting. My father — usually drunk when this happened at that hour — raged at my mother, she would rage back, or sometimes she would cry and beg him be quiet. There were fists pounding on the kitchen table, doors slamming, threats and more shouting. I would lie in my bed, shaking so hard my teeth chattered, scared to death and expecting someone was going to die that night. Or the next time. Or the next one after that. At least on those occasions, I knew I had a reason to be frightened.

I could even understand being afraid and anxious on every one of the many nights when I woke up to the sound of my father being violently sick from drinking. The toilet was just on the other side of the wall beside my bed, and the sounds were so terrifying, I thought he would die.

But I couldn't understand why there were so many times I woke up to absolute silence. The house was dark and still, apart from the occasional quiet hum of the furnace in the basement. And in moments, the shaking and terror would begin, and would continue sometimes for an hour or two until eventually, I fell asleep again, utterly exhausted and having no idea how I would get through school the next day.

In my teens, I developed a phobia about vomiting. I mean, a major phobia. I would have preferred death to vomiting. Seriously. As I had been living in a fairly constant state of anxiety for years, sometimes my stomach would get in such a knot that I felt like I might be sick. This made me even more anxious, which made me feel even more nauseated, and then more fearful that I would be sick — and so on.

Eventually, when it would all subside, I hadn't been sick, and I was back to my usual level of anxiety, I began to fear the next time I'd feel sick, afraid that I might vomit. The whole cycle grew and grew until eventually I was having full-blown panic attacks on a fairly regular basis.

As a child, I would only get them at night. But as a young adult, I began having them during the day, and sometimes in public. The first time was in a supermarket. Suddenly, with no warning and no provocation while I was in the cereal aisle, it started. All by itself, that was alarming and dramatically increased my level of anxiety. It took it to a whole new level. Almost immediately, I became dizzy and thought I might faint. With the development of this new symptom, my anxiety escalated significantly.

I began to fear the supermarket — any supermarket — and got in and out as quickly as possible. Then it happened at the drug store. And at the bank. With each new situation in which I had a panic attack, I'd cross off yet another place on my "safe list." As a single parent, life became extra difficult, as there was no one to do a lot of these things for me.

As often as I could, I would avoid places where I'd had a panic attack. I relied on a couple of friends to do my errands where I could. I stayed home more and more often, fearing more panic attacks in public — which is what agoraphobia is all about. It is not a fear of those places; it is a fear of having a panic attack in one of them.

By then, I was also doing battle with Obsessive Compulsive Disorder (OCD — yet another anxiety disorder). I was terrified of germs and scrubbing my hands countless times every day. I was washing clean dishes before using them and had several other OCD behaviours, too. Dealing with all of this made life as a single parent even more difficult than it needed to be.

To make matters worse, I had also been suffering with anorexia for a few years — nine in all, by the end of it — and spent a good deal of time being anxious, pacing around the kitchen, staring at a tiny amount of food that I knew I had to eat but just couldn't. It might as well have been a plate of poison; I was terrified to eat.

Yet by then, I had two children to take care of and I knew their lives depended on my being okay. For years, I endured one tormented battle after another as the war raged inside me — to eat, or not to eat. I would never wish it on anyone. At 5'9", I weighed approximately 100 lbs. I was a complete and utter mess, to say the least.

I ended up seeing a psychiatrist for some time, but all he did was shove tranquilisers and anti-depressants down my throat, all of which gave me terrible side effects (including more anxiety, of all things...) and none of which helped in the slightest. Eventually, I had the good sense to stop wasting my time in his office.

Somewhere along the way, I heard about an over-the-counter medicine that was used to treat nausea. I figured I ought to try it, as I always got queasy with anxiety or panic attacks — which of course sent me over the edge with my vomiting phobia — and it worked really well.

From that day on, at the first sign of a panic attack and the threat of feeling even a little bit sick, I popped one of those babies. The problem was, as my life was spinning more and more out of control, the anxiety was off the charts. I discovered that these little anti-nausea pills were muscle relaxants, which is why they prevent vomiting. And it didn't take long to figure out that as an added bonus, they eased the anxiety, too.

And with anorexia being an anxiety disorder (although much more complex than that), it meant they could help me eat. I began to pop one just so I could eat a little bit of food without freaking out about it.

Needless to say, I began taking them quite regularly, having been told that they were not physically addictive. Before long, I was making sure there was always a packet in my handbag. I wouldn't go anywhere without them, just in case the anxiety pushed me to the point of feeling sick... I remember driving somewhere once and would be out for most of the evening. I realised I'd taken the pills out of my handbag and had forgotten to put them back. Instantly, I was in a state of panic and had to stop at the nearest drug store to get another packet. I couldn't function without them.

I went on like this for several years, somehow managing to function as a single mum with a job (fortunately I worked from home), until one night when it all caught up with me. It was around 2.00 a.m. and I was desperate for one of my little miracle workers. Heaven only knows how it happened, but I was out of them. I had several of those familiar little boxes, a couple in this dresser, one in that night-stand, another in the medicine cabinet and so on, somehow I'd managed to run out.

I broke into a sweat as I threw a dressing gown around my shoulders and ran down the stairs to get my handbag from the top shelf of the hall closet. Snapping on the light, I plunked my handbag down on a little table by the door and frantically dug for the familiar little box that had saved me every day for the past several years.

As I tore through the contents of my bag, I caught sight of myself in the mirror above the table. I was drawn and pale. There was a frighteningly wild look in my eyes. I looked completely wired, strung out, like a junkie scrambling for her next fix. I stopped cold and stared hard. Shame and self-loathing flooded through every part of my shattered soul. I knew what I had to do.

After six years, it was time to face my addiction. But how? Where would I begin?

This particular drug isn't physically addictive but I was as psychologically addicted as a person can get. My children needed and deserved a whole mother. I swore that although I didn't know how I would do it, I was determined to sort through this nightmare on my own.

As I waded through the mess I'd made, I realised that the only way to get off those pills was to find a way to deal with the anxiety. Having been down the road of useless prescription drugs, it was time to do some research. I found a brilliant little book, "Hope and Help for Your Nerves" by Dr. Claire Weekes. I learned about the mechanics of anxiety and panic attacks, and why the body creates all those scary symptoms like dizziness, tingling in the hands and feet, and a pounding heart that feels like it's going so fast, it will explode. I also learned that it will not. And I learned that although I felt like I would faint, it was only because I was hyperventilating, which also produced the tingling.

The three most important bits of information I learned were

these: Firstly, although in the midst of a panic attack, I was sure I would die, I discovered that I would not.

Secondly, the more I freaked out about how frightening the symptoms were when I was having them, the more anxiety it produced, and of course that made the symptoms worse — and so on.

And thirdly, in between panic attacks, as long as I was worrying about the next one, I was keeping myself "primed and ready" for it because those thoughts would create ongoing anxiety, which made another panic attack all the more likely. In fact, it was pretty much a done deal.

The bottom line was that the more anxious thoughts I had, the more likely I was to have a panic attack. And the more panic attacks I had, the more anxious thoughts I had in between, too. The only way to break the cycle was to stop feeling anxious. If you've ever suffered with anxiety, you know that sounds like it's easier said than done, right? But just because something isn't easy, that doesn't mean it's impossible.

I had found that "first step" in my journey to the moon, and it was really pretty simple. I just had to change my thoughts about what was happening to my body when it was experiencing anxiety and panic. I had to stop fighting it, because the fighting was merely creating more anxiety. The more I became frustrated and agitated about the symptoms, the worse they got.

Instead, I learned to accept whatever my body was feeling and doing, and to tell myself it would pass and I would be okay. I allowed myself to feel fidgety, get up and pace. Sometimes, it helped to play some of my favourite music to distract and calm myself. I had to let my heart race and tell myself that it was okay, it would not explode.

I told myself that these feelings were no big deal, they would pass and I'd be fine. I had to tell myself the dizziness and tingling were because of hyperventilation. I told myself to slow my breathing, I would not faint, and other thoughts such as these.

I had gone off the pills straight away and with my new attitude and approach to the problem, I was astonished by how quickly my anxiety did an about-face. Once I understood what was going on in my body, and that it was made worse by fearing it or fighting it, the general anxiety began to subside right away. Because of that, the number of panic attacks dramatically dropped, too, and when I did have them in those early days and practiced my new way of thinking, they would barely begin before petering out.

So what's this detour got to do with discussing the secret labyrinths of the subconscious?

Everything. It was important to give you a view of how this works, and to offer proof that if you change your thoughts, you can change how you feel. It proves that your thoughts often control what happens in your body, and that your subconsciously-held fears and beliefs will manifest in ways that leave you feeling as though you have no control.

To demonstrate my point, if we go back to my childhood it's easy to see the kinds of thoughts I would have had in such a frightening environment. I was always waiting for the other shoe to drop, wondering when the next attack would be. Whether a physical assault, the mental torment by a sadistic brother, or violation, I was immersed in fearful thoughts.

From my external experiences, my conscious mind gathered information about what I could expect. It used logic and reason to formulate beliefs about myself and the world around me, and deposited them into my subconscious, where they churned up anxiety constantly, whether I was awake or asleep. I believed I wasn't safe. I believed another attack was lurking in the next moment. I believed the world was a frightening place and there was no one to protect me.

Once I began having anxiety disorders and panic attacks, I believed I would die when they became overwhelming. And I believed I was "an anxious person" and that I'd be that way forever. I believed there was no way to change it.

But I was wrong. I began to change my thoughts about that. And over time I had broken the cycle. I was no longer suffering from constant anxiety and frequent eruptions of panic.

This was a brilliant first step for me but I was light years from being fully well. I had yet to uncover so much more that was hiding in the depths of my subconscious in the form of deep-seated beliefs that caused self-destructive behaviours and choices. And then I had to deal with them.

Chapter Seventeen

I t is interesting to me that sometimes we know things even though we do not have any real knowledge or understanding of them.

Take, for example, a Scottish surgeon, who worked in Bengal long before anyone had heard of ether or anaesthetic. Dr James Esdaile had read about mesmerism, a technique which involved repeatedly passing one's hands over a patient's body, but not touching it, coming instead to within about an inch of it.

There was more to it than that, but this rhythmic, repetitious action, done in a darkened room, put people into a state of deep relaxation, a sort of a trance, if you will. It was what we would now call a hypnotic state. He had never actually done it, and although he said, "I shall probably not succeed", he felt compelled to try it on a convict who required surgery, in an effort to reduce or eliminate any sensation of pain during the operation.

Not only was he successful, between 1843 and 1846 he did hundreds of pain-free operations on patients who were awake, including during the removal of malignant tumours, operating on the ears, eyes, and throats, and even doing amputations. The only anaesthetic he used came from the patients' minds.

There were no deaths during the operations, and his post-operative mortality rate was extremely low, approximately 2-3%.

While his patients were in this hypnotic state, Dr Esdaile told them that there would be no sepsis, and in fact most of them had absolutely no infection at all, while a small number had just a minimum.

What makes this even more astonishing is that these surgeries were done well before the discovery of bacteria. People had no knowledge or understanding of the origins of disease or infections, and therefore, they knew nothing about the need for operating in a sterile environment, and with sterile instruments.

Even today, when operations take place in sterile surgical theatres, with medical staff using sterile dressings, antibacterial ointments and so on, infection is still a significant problem. In fact, the Centers for Disease Control in America reported that despite being vigilant about hygiene, MRSA, a bacterial infection that is notorious for springing up in hospitals and nursing homes, was responsible for 94,000 life-threatening infections and over 18,000 deaths in 2005 alone.

Yet in Esdaile's day, operations and recoveries would have taken place in extremely unsanitary surroundings. How was it possible for him to have a nearly non-existent infection rate?

It is because he was directly accessing the subconscious minds of the patients and depositing new thoughts, which they accepted and believed. Those new thoughts created all the necessary neurotransmitters, sent out all the right messages to every cell in their bodies, and put the immune system on high alert for any invaders to be eliminated immediately.

Consciously, these patients knew nothing about the cause of infection. Yet subconsciously, they had effectively commanded their bodies to do what was necessary to ensure there would be no infection. Against all odds, given the terribly unsanitary conditions, there was virtually none.

In the same way, their thoughts had created chemical messages that told their bodies they would not experience any pain. Wide awake and enduring amputations and all manner of invasive surgeries, these patients felt nothing.

You can see by this example how powerful our thoughts are, and therefore, how powerful the subconscious is. For what else is the subconscious, but our thoughts playing over and over again in the form of beliefs that have been planted there? The brain is a visible, photographable tangible thing, but it is not the mind, which is intangible and cannot be seen. Invisible though it may be, it is nevertheless very real, an electromagnetic field of energy, creativity and possibility.

You may be wondering, perhaps a bit nervously, how can someone such as Dr Esdaile, or indeed, any hypnotist, so easily plant ideas into the minds of others. As a hypnotist, I have often heard such concerns, especially because of stage shows in which people are "made" to do ridiculous things whilst in a hypnotic state. If it is really so simple to access the subconscious and make people believe whatever the hypnotist suggests, is this not dangerous? Isn't it possible, then, that they could be made to do things that go completely against what they believe?

The answer is no. And the reason is very simple, yet most reassuring. It is because of the conscious mind, or as I like to call it, the Gatekeeper. The subject must accept a suggestion by the hypnotist in order for it to have any effect at all, and those people who do goofy things on stage have done so because in the interests of having fun, they agreed to those suggestions while in a hypnotic state.

The first misconception about hypnosis is that subjects are asleep or unconscious, and completely unaware of what is happening. The second is that the hypnotist has any control over the subject.

In our normal, waking lives, there is essentially a wall between the conscious and the subconscious minds. If not for that wall, we would constantly be bombarded with memories, fears, thoughts about everything that has ever happened to us. It would be truly over-whelming.

Therefore, most of our experiences get locked away in that labyrinth, where it looks after them for us, while the conscious mind goes about its daily activities, taking in what's happening to us and around us, giving us the information we need to get on with the business of living.

Hypnosis is merely a deep state of relaxation, during which that wall between the conscious and subconscious comes down, allowing thought, memories and so on to flow freely back and forth between them. Subjects are awake and aware of their surroundings. Far from being asleep, they are hyper focused on what's happening. In fact, the more relaxed the subjects, the more heightened their senses become. The more deeply they allow themselves to relax, the better the suggestions work. But not without the approval of the conscious mind.

Ever vigilant, it is there, watching the proceedings, the Gate-keeper, protecting the subject from harm. When a suggestion is given, the conscious mind is there, listening intently, hearing every word and deciding whether or not it is acceptable. If so, it deposits it into the subconscious. If not, the suggestion is simply rejected and has no effect.

For example, since I began using hypnosis as a part of my coun-selling work in the mid-'90s, I've helped numerous people stop smok-ing. All of them stopped after no more than two sessions. All of them, that is, but one. This woman had come to me *only* because her family had insisted, and there she sat in my office, angry, arms folded, obvious hostile. She squinted at me and fairly hissed her monosyl-labic answers to my questions. There was no part of her that wanted to stop smoking. She didn't care about the smell, the cost, the health issues; there was no motivation whatsoever.

Because subjects have to agree to suggestions in order for them to work, hypnotists have absolutely no control over their minds whatsoever. Therefore, I was certain that this woman would not even enter a hypnotic state. Although she agreed to lie back in the recliner opposite me and close her eyes, no doubt that with every suggestion I gave to relax, visualise this sunny beach or that fluffy little cloud, she was sullenly thinking, "NO! I WON'T!"

And you can forget any of the suggestions I gave about not smoking. If I told her that all cravings for cigarettes had vanished, she would be thinking, "NO! They haven't! I love my cigarettes!" If anything, hypnosis had probably only served to make her love smoking even more — if that was possible.

And of course, no doubt she left my office, got into her car and smoked her brains out all the way home. But at least she could tell her family, "There! I went! And SEE?? It didn't work! Now leave me alone!" In retrospect, I should have refused to do the treatment. She insisted, but I should have just said no. Ah... live and learn, right?!

So yes, it's true that the subconscious is responsible for our choices and our emotions, but only because of what we allow ourselves to think about and believe. When we decide to pay attention to why we make our choices, and why we feel the way we do about things, sometimes we realise that our old beliefs don't work for us any more.

Hypnosis is just one way (the "fast track"!) that we can effectively get into the subconscious with a screwdriver and a pair of pliers, tinker around a bit and presto! The result is a change in behaviour, the release of old "stuff" or long-standing fears. But not because the subconscious has made the decision. The Gatekeeper does that. The subconscious is only responding to what it has been fed. If you want a different result, you have to feed it a new diet.

While I was going through this whole self-healing experiment, I had a hypnosis client who had come to me to stop smoking (and yep, he actually wanted it!). Not wanting to cause any harm while gently treading through his vulnerable subconscious mind, I knew I had to choose my words carefully. I was mindful not to use any negatives, because the subconscious does not recognise them.

135

For example, I couldn't say, "You won't want to smoke" because the subconscious would only hear "You want to smoke." Of course, I've known this since becoming a hypnotist in the mid-'90s, but as I was in the midst of my own self-healing and the research that would ultimately become this book.

As I sat with him, carefully choosing my words to avoid the negative ones, suddenly, I had a huge "Aha!" moment. You know, one of those big, bright halogen lights that goes on over your head? Yeah, one of those.

It was so simple, and so profound at the same time: The subconscious does not accept negatives. **The subconscious does not accept negatives!** It's like our 'default' setting is about positivity, right down to this very deep level of our awareness and our 'being-ness', but I'd never thought about it before.

I'm certainly thinking about it now. We're used to being ill now and then; we think it's normal. But that doesn't mean it's *supposed* to be a part of our existence. It's not our natural state to be ill. It's not normal. We're designed for positive environments and energy, which is where we thrive and do well.

Negative energy makes us sick. Negative thoughts make us depressed, sad etc. — and these emotions make us sick, too. Everything negative is meant to be unacceptable, damaging and destructive to us; we are not designed to tolerate it, and it is *not even in the vocabulary of the subconscious.*

And the subconscious is the storehouse for all of our experiences; it is the powerhouse that creates illness or wellness in response to what our conscious minds feed it. The fact that it cannot digest negative words speaks volumes about our inherent inability to thrive or grow or even survive on anything other than positivity.

Even Hippocrates seemed to understand this nearly 2,500 years ago. Doctors were told to keep examining rooms well lit and cheerful, as he believed that it would hasten the healing process if patients were in good spirits.

One of the most convincing and curious aspects of hypnosis, or to be more precise, of the subconscious, is post-hypnotic suggestion. As the name implies, it is a suggestion that is meant to have an effect after the subject is no longer in hypnosis. It's useful if, for example, you're being treated for your fear of dentistry. Been there, done that. I was that patient. And all I can say is, thank heaven for having found a dentist who used hypnosis! His post-hypnotic suggestions stuck. I haven't feared dentistry in 40 years.

If you go prior to your appointment, while in a hypnotic state you'll likely be given suggestions about being relaxed and sleeping well the night before dental appointments. You may be told that when the dental chair goes back and the light goes on over your head, you'll relax deeply and will be quite happy to let the dentist do his work.

Later, during appointments when you're having work done, you won't actually be hypnotised but these suggestions will still work because they were planted in the subconscious during a hypnotic state.

At the Foothills Hospital in Calgary, I used to teach classes for expectant parents on how to use hypnosis during childbirth. In an effort to reassure nervous couples that hypnosis could work miracles for labouring women, I would always do a quick yet powerful demonstration of post-hypnotic suggestion.

Bear in mind, as I've said already, that my suggestions would only work if they were acceptable to the subjects. I put the whole class into hypnosis, then gave the suggestion that everyone's right hand would become completely numb, as though it had been shot full of novocaine. I told them that when they came out of hypnosis, the numbness would remain, and they would transfer that numbness to their jaws by gently rubbing the area.

Then I would bring them out of hypnosis, encourage them to transfer that numbness, and wait to see what happened. Within a few minutes of rubbing their jaws, everyone felt something happening. Some said their lips or jaws felt a bit thick, others said they were completely numb in those areas, while still others sounded like they'd just been to the dentist as they announced (with some difficulty!) that their tongues were also numb.

No matter how often I did this to rooms full of people, it never ceased to amaze me just how powerful the subconscious is. Yet there is another incredible trick of the mind that is so shocking, so intriguing, and so mysterious, every time I think about it, I continue to be fascinated, as it is among the most astonishing phenomena in the world. It proves beyond any shadow of a doubt that the mind is capable of creating — and destroying — diseases or disorders at will.

Chapter Eighteen

I'd like to introduce you to a young woman called Jenny. She is 23, and aside from English, she speaks fluent French, German and Italian. She is extremely bright and well spoken, and loves her job as a teacher. She has terrible allergies to almost everything, so her diet is extremely restricted. She goes into anaphylactic shock if she eats shellfish or nuts of any kind. She never touches a drop of alcohol, as even a very small amount of it will make her violently ill.

Now meet Caroline. She is 52. She suffers from severe depression, tends to make half-hearted attempts at suicide and has no confidence whatsoever. Timid as a mouse, she is quiet when in the company of others. She has a serious sweet tooth and particularly loves pecan pie as often as she can get it. She has frightening scars from burns on her arms, which she usually hides under long sleeves. They are a painful reminder of her very abusive mother.

Then there is Tom. He's 17, a high school dropout with bad skin, and a ton of rage. He's always threatening to hit people, and sometimes follows through and does it. He drinks too often and too much, occasionally to the point of passing out. Never a good student, he can barely read.

And there is Helen. A shy but friendly 32-year-old mother, whose doctor has recently discovered a tumour on her liver. She has a lot of trouble with insomnia, and takes strong sleeping pills to get through the night sometimes.

Last but not least, there is little Suzy. She is 5, very talkative and loves to climb up into people's laps and be cuddled. Usually, she smells of peanut butter, as it is her favourite thing in the world and she's always got a bit of it on one cheek or the other.

Now imagine that all of these people - and more - are all rolled up into one physical body. Yes, I am talking about Dissociative Identity Disorder (DID), previously known as Multiple Personality Disorder. In a very small percentage of individuals who have endured extreme abuse or trauma, somehow the mind creates several completely separate identities in what is believed to be an intriguing attempt to divide up and dole out the emotional pain, which is far more than one individual could bear.

This, in and of itself, is amazing. Although all of them exist in the same body, each of the personalities, called "alters", has completely different brain waves from the others. Their handwriting is unique from one another, too, so that analysts think samples came from separate individuals.

There can be both male and female alters in the same body, and they can all have different results from one another on IQ tests. Some may speak foreign languages and write poetry, while others may be illiterate. Their voices sound different from one another, their speech and mannerisms change from one alter to the next. Some of the alters need glasses, whilst others may have extraordinarily good vision.

As interesting as all of this is, it is not the astonishing "trick of the mind" to which I was referring. It is not the absolute proof that I said exists regarding our ability to create or destroy diseases or disorders. That proof lies in the example I gave above, with five separate personalities who exist in the same body, yet each one has specific ailments or physical conditions that the others do not.

Jenny's allergies are dreadful during times when she is the alter who is in control, becoming anaphylactic with nuts, but as soon as the next one takes over, the allergies disappear. Caroline loves her pecan pie; Suzy adores peanut butter on toast. They do not suffer any adverse reaction, much less life-threatening anaphylaxis, from eating nuts.

And if Jenny steps in as the controlling alter during one of Tom's drunken evenings, she will not become ill or feel the effects of the alcohol at all — because she does not drink it. Even though it is the same alcohol-infused blood that courses through that physical body, Jenny believes she is a completely separate person, and as such, she cannot feel the alcohol because she did not consume it.

Helen visits the doctor, wearing short sleeves that show off her soft, smooth skin, but shortly after she views the X-ray of the tumour on her liver, Caroline takes control and ends up in hospital after smashing her car in a suicide attempt. When her abdomen is X-rayed, there is no trace of the tumour on her liver. But they do find burn scars on her arms...

Although I made up these personalities, they are based on documented evidence about people with DID. In one physical body, depending on which alter is in control, burns, scars, tumours, cysts, allergies, diabetes, epilepsy, and all sorts of other ailments come and go, come and go, almost in the blink of an eye as the alters switch from one to the next. If one is intoxicated but another takes over, the second one will not feel the alcohol because he or she did not consume it. A woman with DID may even have two or three menstrual periods in a month, as her alters will have different cycles from one another.

We can read about these cases and simply stop at thinking about how incredible they are, and what a marvel and a mystery the human mind is. Or we can move one step beyond and realise what is happening in these people, and why these phenomena can even occur. It's because of the power in their minds.

There's no physical explanation for the repeated disappearance and reappearance of burns, scars or tumours, or for any of the other incredible physical changes, disorders or diseases that are found amongst alters in people with DID. It's entirely a construct of the mind. It is the power that comes from belief, from thoughts creating chemical messages that are sent out in an instant to every single cell in the body. And those cells respond immediately in people with DID because the belief of each alter is so strong.

Caroline was the alter whose arms were burned by her mother. She remembers it, and of course there are scars. But Helen was not burned, nor Tom, nor Suzy, nor Jenny, nor any of the others that might exist in my fictional DID patient. Because each one of them is as real and distinct as you and I are from one another, when any one of them other than Caroline steps in and takes control, those scars cannot, should not, must not and will not be there, because those people were not burned.

They believe they are as separate from one another as you and I are, and therefore, it wouldn't even cross their minds that they should share scars, tumours, etc. To them, that is just as impossible as it is for you to share the long scar on my right leg, a remnant from a nasty incident with a barbed-wire fence when I was nine.

Equally fascinating is the fact that people with DID do not age as quickly as "normal" individuals, and they heal much faster, too. Even third degree burns heal at an astonishing rate. There are documented cases of people with DID who have one alter in particular who is focused on nothing but healing, using visualising, meditation or whatever other methods he or she believes are necessary.

It's thought that even when an alter isn't "up front" as the controlling personality, he or she in the background, awake and functional, if not outwardly obvious. So it's quite possible to have at least one alter visualing healing round the clock. The rest of us don't have the luxury of spending 24 hours a day focusing on healing ourselves, but an alter of someone with DID does. This would certainly account for the rapidity of their healing, as well as the fact that they age slower than the rest of us.

When we consider that these people are able to create tumours or "delete" them, and re-create them over and over again, although we may understand the mechanics of this in terms of belief and the body's response, we may wonder, "How is it so easy for them? Why can't I do it like that?"

It's all down to strength of belief, really. As previously stated, alters see themselves just as real and as separate as you and I are. Therefore, when an alter steps into the control position, the belief in that identity is just as strong as your belief that you are not me, and the physical body must respond to the thoughts. But you see, we tell ourselves "I have a tumour! Oh I hope I can make it go away but I don't really know if I can! That's impossible, isn't it? I'll try..." and so on, with doubt being the culprit in either slowing, or halting the healing process.

I can understand now why I had so much success with the affirmations I used for my ailments (eg. hip, knee and heart while going for walks, or the hot flushes of menopause). Although the problems didn't disappear overnight, there was a dramatic improvement rather quickly, which continued over the weeks that followed as I kept up with these "conversations". It is well worth the bit of time and effort it takes to use this technique.

Just think: If we were able to believe that we're perfectly healed, and believe it with just as much strength and conviction as the alters of people with DID believe in the conditions of "their" bodies, then our ailments would vanish just as quickly as theirs do when another alter steps in.

In these kinds of situations, there is a direct relationship between beliefs and their ability to create change in a body. "I believe I have a tumour" — and presto, there it is. And of course, there's another way that beliefs can alter physical health and even cause death. People who believe they're failures, or that the world or their families would be better off without them, or who believe there is no other solution to terrible problems can end up attempting suicide. If they survive, they may end up with long-term or permanent damage to their bodies or minds, depending on what method they used. At worst, they may succeed and end their lives. And all because of what they believed.

There is a less direct way that beliefs can affect physical health, even to the point of causing death, and that's with eating disorders. Anorexia and bulimia have nothing to do with food or with appetite but they have everything to do with self-image, self-worth, self-esteem, and issues of control. These illnesses are complex with various factors causing them, and are often driven by a need to be perfect, which stems from a belief in being inadequate, not good enough, or unloved. Those beliefs can cause death in up to 20% of the victims of these disorders.

In fact, anorexia kills more young women aged 15-24 than all other causes of death combined.

This is a frightening statistic, especially when you consider that it is based purely on what these young women believe about themselves, their relationships, their circumstances — beliefs that will have been the result of other people's opinions of them, other people's treatment of them, and will not be based on reality.

Those toxic, negative opinions are all about the people who are offering them and have nothing to do with anyone on the receiving end. If people with eating disorders could just change their thoughts, and ultimately their self-destructive beliefs, they would survive — and be well.

That old saying, "It's all in your head" is far more truthful than we realise. Unfortunately, it's cursed with a derogatory connotation, as though we are mentally or emotionally weak if our thoughts are seen to be causing any sort of illness.

Likewise with the placebo effect in terms of it making us well, although for centuries we have been aware of its power. For how many decades have we been giggling to ourselves about all those poor suckers in drug trials who have ended up thinking they felt better, when all they got was a little sugar pill? We snicker and think, "How foolish they are! Guess they were never really sick in the first place!" — because it was all in their heads, right?

Wrong.

We were the ones being foolish. Rather than understanding, embracing and learning to use the power of the mind, we ridiculed it and made light of it when we could have been using it to our benefit all this time.

Of people who have had a placebo "painkiller", 30-60% will have relief. Why the success? How does it work? The subjects believe they have taken something that will remove their pain; they expect the pain to disappear. Their thoughts, therefore, create matching chemical messengers, in the form of endorphins, and these messengers are sent out into the body, where receptors are waiting for them. Subjects do not merely imagine that their pain had vanished; they create endorphins, the body's natural pain relievers.

We see proof of this in a subsequent study, which Deepak Chopra discusses in his book, *Quantum Healing*. naloxone is a drug that knocks out the effects of morphine. Therefore, if someone has taken morphine for pain relief, then receives a dose of naloxone, the morphine no longer works and the pain returns.

Interestingly, when a placebo had brought relief from pain, and those subjects were given a dose of naloxone, their pain returned just as surely as if they'd had morphine. This suggests that endorphins had actually been created and delivered to receptors. It also suggests that endorphins and morphine must be essentially the same drug.

Results varied both in pain relief with the placebo, and the return of pain with a dose of naloxone. As with any type of treatment for pain, whether with drugs, acupuncture, homeopathy or hypnosis, results can never be guaranteed.

Why the variation in results? No doubt scientists and researchers would have a whole list of possible answers to that, and we know there isn't only one that is correct. I believe that at least to a large extent, it is due to the dubiousness of hope and doubt versus the absolutes of belief, expectation and trust. As I've already explained, changes in health on any level, for better or worse, seem dependent upon strength of belief.

In researching this book, I was reminded of thousands of years' healing done by religious leaders, medicine men, and so on. Through the ages, there have been numerous accounts of dramatic healing taking place as a result of priests or other religious leaders performing rituals and saying prayers over the sick. It was —and still is, for many - believed that healing came from God (or "gods" or "spirits" etc.). Therefore, any such healing could happen only if people had faith and a belief in God's existence and ability to heal.

Numerous cultures have been very spiritually based, with all conditions and circumstances of life being due to God's will, God's wrath, God's happiness or other desires or emotional responses. Since ancient times he has been seen to punish or reward individuals or whole communities for their actions - or their inactions. For thousands of years, people have believed that God is omniscient, omnipresent and most importantly, omnipotent.

It is this belief in the power of God that is the basis for the acceptance that he can heal — if he so chooses — and if that understanding is accompanied by certain rituals and prayers. Therefore, when all conditions are met, there isn't just the hope, there is the certainty that a healing will take place. And it does.

One has only to look at modern-day snake-handling Christians to find an example of just how people continue to tie faith and belief to health and healing. Originating in Appalachia in the eastern U.S. in the early 1900s, the practice consists of singing and dancing whilst holding a venomous snake, passing it from one person to another and risking a deadly bite. Occasionally, it can also involve the consumption of strychnine or other poisons. Despite being outlawed in various parts of the country, many rural churches still conduct regular services that include these activities.

Based on two Biblical passages, it is believed that performing these acts is a test of one's faith in God. First, from Luke 10:19, "I have given you authority to trample on snakes and scorpions and to overcome all the power of the enemy; nothing will harm you." Secondly, from Mark 16:18, which says, "They shall take up serpents; and if they drink any deadly thing, it shall not hurt them..."

These people believe that whatever happens as a result of drinking poison or being bitten by a venomous snake, it is God's will. Should they become ill, they do not seek medical attention and instead rely on prayer, which, more often than not, is successful and they recover. However, many have died but this doesn't frighten those who pursue these activities because they believe that their faith in God will grant them eternal salvation, which is of the utmost importance to them. As far as they're concerned, living or dead, it's all good.

Interestingly, although they will not seek medical treatment as a result of their poison-drinking and snake-handling, they will for other ailments that are not related to testing their faith in God.

While writing this book and researching the powerful effects of belief on healing, I was met with what I thought was a flaw in the theory. I was thinking about all those years when I was suffering with my heart problem and trigeminal neuralgia to the point that I became suicidal. Not only had I witnessed some pretty remarkable healing results in myself, my family, friends, and patients using homeopathy, its philosophy is sound. It has been well proven round the world, beginning in the last 1700s. I had every reason to believe that it would cure me. I thought it was the magic bullet for everyone and everything in terms of its healing ability.

With such a firm belief in the potential for homeopathy to cure me, why, then, did the placebo effect not come into play and "override" the lack of results from taking incorrect remedies?

If the placebo effect is about believing that you have taken something that will absolutely make you well, why didn't that belief work when I was 100% convinced that homeopathy would cure me? Especially when I had taken the remedy that was selected by the brilliant principal of the School of Homeopathy, a man I admired and respected and in whose abilities I had the utmost confidence? Shouldn't my firm belief in homeopathy have healed me on any one of those occasions, due to the placebo effect, when I had taken a remedy that had had little or no effect?

As I considered how this might affect my entire theory about the relationship between self-healing and the power of belief, I realised why the placebo effect had not picked up where homeopathy had left off. It had nothing to do with my belief in the principles of homeopathy. It had everything to do with knowing very well that achieving a cure depends upon finding the correct remedy; therefore, every one of them was taken with a big question mark.

To make matters worse, I was well aware of how complicated it can be to find the correct remedy, and because of my chaotic and tumultuous life and decades of ill health, my case was complex. This made it impossible to be certain of a remedy's success. It was always a "cross your fingers and hope for the best" scenario, and probably with a much bigger dose of doubt than was helpful, especially as time went on and I lost more and more hope. I had almost given up entirely so that every time I tried another remedy, I was often thinking it probably wouldn't work.

The correct prescription would not be affected by my doubts, fears and growing hopelessness, but the placebo effect would. Remedies work on babies, animals, people who are in comas. They work on people who "don't believe in homeopathy." But a placebo's effectiveness relies solely on a firm belief in its ability to heal.

We have established the powerful link between our thoughts, the energy they produce to create chemical messages, and how the physical body is affected. And it's clear that the strength of our thoughts and conviction of our beliefs influences how much and how quickly we can bring about physical changes — for better or for worse.

But just what is a thought? And why it is so powerful?

Chapter Nineteen

There's still a lot we don't understand about the brain or the human mind, but we can make some pretty good guesses based on what we do know.

First, it helps to be crystal clear about the difference between the two. The **brain** is a physical, mechanical organ — a real, tangible part of the body that handles speech, writing, memory and countless other functions. It has no consciousness of its own, no will, no emotions.

The **mind**, on the other hand, is completely intangible. You can't see it or point to a specific spot in the brain where it "lives." It's your thoughts, your intellect, your consciousness — and your subconsciousness. It's the managing director, the choreographer, the conductor of the whole orchestra that is your body. This is your own infinite creative intelligence working hand in hand with your physical self. Whether you realise it or not, the mind and body are constantly sending messages back and forth, checking in with each other about what's going on.

As I've mentioned before, thoughts show up as electromagnetic waves, which can be picked up on an EEG. Half the energy of these waves is carried by the electric field and the other half by the magnetic field. And since energy can't be created or destroyed, the energy from those waves has to go somewhere — it appears to be used by, or spread throughout, the body.

The electrical currents inside us (and in all living organisms) are known as **bioelectricity**. They occur when chemical energy is converted to electrical energy. Many different biological processes generate these currents, which cells then use to send impulses along nerve fibres, regulate muscle contraction, and control metabolism. These impulses can vary widely from one organism to another — anywhere from a single millivolt to several hundred.

In the human body, three main types of electrical signals have been identified:

- the electrical waves in the brain, measured on an electroencephalogram (EEG);
- the electrical impulses created by the heart muscle's contractions, which show up on an electrocardiogram (ECG) and are about 100 times stronger than brain waves;
- and the surface electrical potential, which is measurable on the skin.

That last one — the heart's electrical signal being as strong as the skin's surface potential — is especially interesting. Its origin and full significance are still unknown, but it's widely used in psychological research because it's highly sensitive to emotional and physiological changes. The skin's bioelectrical conductivity shifts with hydration, stress, emotions and disease.

So yes, it's fair to say we're bioelectric beings. But it's probably even more accurate to call us **bioelectromagnetic** creatures — living organisms who produce electromagnetic fields. Our cells use bioelectricity to store metabolic energy, which powers their many tasks and allows them to communicate with one another. Bioelectromagnetism is simply the electrical currents and magnetic fields produced by an organism. All living things have it — even plants. Some animals, like sharks and migratory birds, seem to use the Earth's magnetic field as a kind of compass, while others, like eels, can generate electric fields outside their bodies.

Now that we know we're bio-electromagnetic beings, it's no surprise that people have been tinkering with ways to measure and use that energy for decades. Enter biofeedback machines. They can monitor muscle action, skin temperature, skin electrical activity, heart and brain activity — you name it. These devices have been used to help diagnose conditions, and also to treat anxiety, migraines, pain and a long list of other common complaints.

We already know that disturbances in the body's bioelectrical system can cause a huge range of diseases and disorders. Think about it: polio and ALS attack motor neurons; herniated discs in the spine interfere with nerve roots; and countless infectious, metabolic and inflammatory conditions damage peripheral nerves. All of these are usually chalked up to "physical causes." A doctor might even hum the old children's song while explaining it: "the leg bone's connected to the ankle bone..." But when the flow of bioelectrical communication from one part of the body to another is interrupted, something goes haywire — and we think that's the whole story.

But here's the rub: can doctors explain why the skin's electrical conductivity changes with emotions and stress? Can they tell us exactly why blood pressure and heart rate jump when someone's angry? They'll say, correctly, that certain chemicals or hormones are released — the fight-or-flight response and so on. But can they explain precisely how an emotion sparks such a chain of events? No. They can only say that it happens.

At first glance, it seems as though our emotions are in charge — like they have a will of their own and can direct everything, right down to the invisible bioelectrical currents on the skin, measurable only with specialised equipment. But that's not quite it. Our emotions don't actually drive our bodies to function or respond the way they do. As I explained earlier, it's our **thoughts** that sit in the driver's seat. Now you can see the next step: our emotions are the petrol. They provide the energy that fuels the physical responses, the release of chemical messengers, and so on. What you think creates what you feel, and that emotion then becomes the driving force that tells your body what to do.

I'm reminded of my fourth pregnancy. I was never what you'd call "a natural" at labour and delivery — my experiences had always been long, miserable, and topped off with life-threatening post-partum haemorrhages. I was dreading another ordeal. Because hypnosis had helped me with other problems, I decided to try it for childbirth. So off I went to see a well-known hypnotist in Calgary, hoping for some post-hypnotic suggestion that would keep me calm and able to cope with the pain.

While in a fairly light state of hypnosis, I remember him connecting a feedback thermometer to my lower back and asking me to imagine the area getting very warm. I pictured myself sitting on a hearth with my bare back to a roaring fire. I could almost feel the heat, and in my mind I could see the glow in a darkened room. Within minutes, he became very excited — I'd managed to move the temperature gauge a few degrees Celsius, further than anyone he'd ever seen.

Then he told me to make my back cold. So I imagined lying naked on my back in a snowbank (at seven months pregnant, this was quite the comic mental picture!). In a few moments, the gauge shifted again — this time a few degrees in the opposite direction. He asked me to make it warm again, and once more I got the same quick response.

I was astonished at the time, but I didn't fully appreciate how amazing it was until I started researching for this book. When you look at how complex our bodies are, it's incredible — and yet, in a way, it's so simple. Just by directing our thoughts, by choosing what to picture and focus on, we can influence the body's energy and its processes. Truly incredible.

While researching for this book, I came across a lot of information about so-called "spontaneous cures" of cancer. In *Quantum Healing*, Deepak Chopra mentions studies in the U.S. and Japan in which almost every patient reports a powerful shift in awareness — a "knowing" that they will be healed. These patients describe reaching a new level of consciousness where cancer simply does not exist.

Once they reach that level of understanding, cancer cells sometimes disappear rapidly — even quite literally overnight. In other cases the cells stabilise and, although they may not vanish, they cause no further damage. Chopra also refers to another cancer study in which people recovered from late-stage, metastasised cancer using positive emotions, while others with small tumours and early diagnoses died after sinking into negative emotions. He tells of a man who had a tumour on his lung for years and it remained unchanged — until he was told it was probably cancer. Within three months of hearing that news, it changed rapidly and took his life.

Clearly our thoughts produce astonishing amounts of energy. We already know from Chapter 3 that a thought is a measurable electromagnetic wave with the power to create chemical messengers that didn't exist before that thought arose.

One afternoon, while reflecting on all this, I stumbled onto the next piece of this remarkable puzzle. I was having my usual healing meditation — something I do while soaking in a candlelit bath — when I remembered hearing about a Japanese researcher, Dr. Masaru Emoto. He had discovered that water is affected by energy, as if it has a kind of consciousness. I didn't know much about it, only that it involved writing words so the water could "see" them, and supposedly the water would take on the energy of those words.

That gave me an idea. Shortly afterwards, I put a small selection of river stones in my bathtub, each one inscribed with words such as love, patience, joy, peace, perfect health. From then on, my bathing meditations reached a whole other level. I wasn't just doing a healing meditation while soaking in hot water anymore; I was actively visualising the energy of each word infusing the water itself, then flowing through me and making me well.

I noticed a real difference in how I felt during and after those meditations. Whether it was the meditation alone, the hope, the positive energy of the experience, or something truly altering my energy and therefore my body, I'll never know. But I did — and still do — love my bathing meditations, and I deeply appreciate how wonderful they make me feel.

I felt Dr. Emoto's work deserved a closer look. I began by searching for information and photographs online and ended up buying a couple of his books. What I discovered was far more incredible than I could have imagined — and it took my self-healing project to a whole new level, forever changing many aspects of my life for the better.

Chapter Twenty

Since the 1990s, Dr. Emoto has travelled the world, giving talks and showing slides of ice crystals he said were shaped by energy and emotion. His work has been criticised by scientists, but there are many possible reasons why they might not appreciate his dramatic results. Still, that doesn't make them any less real — or any less valid.

The short version of Dr. Emoto's work is this: he placed a jar of water between two speakers and played classical music so that the sound waves would essentially pass through the water. When he froze the water and photographed the ice crystals, they were absolutely stunning. He tried again using heavy metal music, and the ice crystals turned into a terrible, splattered, chaotic mess. These tests, and others like them, were repeated over and over, and the results were always the same.

Next, he experimented with written words, taping them to jars so the words faced the water. Words like "Gratitude," "Thank you" and "I love you" produced perfect, stunning crystals, while "You make me sick! I'll kill you!" and "You fool!" left splattered messes like the ones exposed to angry heavy metal music. Again and again, his team got consistent results, producing tens of thousands of slides using words and music.

Sometimes the ice crystals even reflected the character of the words or music. "You're cute" produced a crystal that did, indeed, look "cute." When Emoto played "Heartbreak Hotel," the crystal split into two parts — like a broken heart. And when he played Bach's *Goldberg Variations*, the ice crystals looked very much like the ones from the word "Gratitude." That's especially interesting because Bach wrote that music out of gratitude for the person for whom it was named. It was as though the water felt the energy of gratitude Bach had put into the music and mirrored it in the crystals.

Clearly, Dr. Emoto's work shows that the crystalline structure of water can be altered depending on the energy, or vibrational frequency, it's exposed to.

As I thought about his findings, I remembered something I'd been told at a homeopathy workshop many years earlier — something I'd quietly thought was questionable at best. The instructor described how a patient once rang him from a distant, snowbound mountain cabin. Her child was seriously ill and she couldn't get out for medicine. After she gave all the symptoms, the instructor selected a remedy, which she didn't have on hand. He told her to write the name of the remedy on a piece of paper, put it under a glass of water (preferably in sunlight for a few hours), then give her child a spoonful of it. We were told it worked.

I've had my share of unusual experiences, but even so, I raised a very sceptical eyebrow at that story.

Yet after reading about Dr. Emoto's work, it started to make sense. Really, I had no business doubting it, given what I already knew about how homeopathic remedies are created — and why people think they're just sugar pills. Remedies are made by taking a substance found in nature, making a tincture of it, then diluting it repeatedly in a specific way so that eventually no actual molecules of the original substance remain. What you get is its pure energy. It's not a physical substance; it's what we call "energetic medicine," like acupuncture or reiki, and it doesn't interfere with drugs a patient might be taking.

The water "remembers" the information it has been given and "copies" it with each dilution. It's a lot like new cells copying information from the ones they're replacing. DNA is obviously crucial to that process, but I'd suggest the water content in the cells also plays a part, giving us a chance to change the information new cells receive as they form.

Again, I'm giving you the view of the forest rather than the trees, but the point is this: I had studied homeopathy at length and understood the science behind it — which is far more detailed than I've outlined here. The short version is that it depends on the memory of water. I'd just never thought about it quite like that before.

Now, adding Dr. Emoto's work into the mix — showing that water retains the energy and feeling of the words it's been "shown" — it suddenly made perfect sense to me that the woman stuck on the side of a mountain with her sick child could have found healing for him in such a peculiar way.

I've always been curious, and thinking about all this gave me an idea for an experiment early on in my self-healing project. One morning, I filled a glass jug with water and wrote "joy" and "peace" on a piece of paper, sticking it to the side of the jar with the words facing inward. I wondered if it would have any effect on me — and if so, what that might be. I left it for a few hours and went about my day, then later began drinking the water as I normally would. I honestly didn't expect anything to happen. This was one big "unknown," and, if I'm truthful, I found it hard to believe I'd feel any different as a result of this experiment — certainly not right away. I figured if anything changed, it would take days. And, frankly, I felt a bit silly even doing it. But no one had to know, right? So I carried on with my day, sipping a glass every hour or two.

It was a busy day, but a few hours in, I stopped for a late-afternoon break. With my mind out of work mode, I couldn't help but notice that the debilitating homesickness I'd been living with had shifted. For the first time since moving back to Canada, that awful black cloud had lifted a little. I actually felt happy and somewhat content. I can't say the homesickness was gone, but I was no longer drowning in it.

Frankly, I don't believe it will ever go completely. I fell in love with England long ago, moved there, became a British citizen, and in every way that matters it is still my home. But at least now I could function without bursting into tears at the very thought of it. Not every thought was a painful, wistful wish anymore. Sometimes I could even smile fondly as I remembered it.

Over the next several days, I kept refilling the jug, drinking in the energy of "joy" and "peace" several times a day. I had to admit I felt calmer and happier in general. And if I'm honest, a part of me didn't want to feel that way, because it felt disloyal to England and to the people I love there. It was as though being happy or at peace about Calgary meant my love for my home and my English "family" had somehow diminished.

Then suddenly, a light went on. I realised I could make peace with living in Calgary — at least for now — without it taking away anything from my love for England or the people I left behind. I'd given myself permission to be happy, and that was a gigantic step.

I knew it was possible this shift was just a coincidence, but that seemed highly unlikely given my long-standing feelings about leaving England and about living in Calgary. I also knew the improvement might be the placebo effect, and that would have been fine with me too. As I discussed back in Chapter 18, the placebo effect is far from something to sneer at; it's a powerful healing tool. Results are results, however they're achieved. More importantly, the placebo effect validates the whole point of this book: healing begins with what we believe and the thoughts we generate.

Still, on the chance that my experiment really had worked on a physical and energetic level, I decided it was worth tackling something specific and trying again.

Next on my list was the bane of my existence — the desire to smoke. For the most part, I wasn't giving in to the urge and only had a couple of cigarettes while in the occasional company of the few smokers I knew. But in between visits, the craving could be agonising.

I was fed up with battling the issue for years and detested the hypocrisy of it. I just wanted it gone from my life. I'd done enough soul-searching and self-analysis over the years to understand that smoking was a self-destructive response to issues going back to my earliest existence. Although I'd made a lot of progress healing those wounds, something was still stuck and causing me grief. Deep inside, that emotionally abandoned baby girl didn't feel as though she deserved to live, and so she sabotaged my efforts to be well. She didn't feel loved, valued or accepted.

As an unborn baby, she knew everyone but her mother wanted her aborted. She felt her mother's love, but there was far more fear and rejection from others. Against her mother's will, the baby was eventually taken from her and put into foster care. Not understanding the separation, the baby believed she was not lovable, that her mother didn't want her — even though that wasn't true. Later, after leaving foster care and being adopted, things got worse. The tiny girl quickly realised she'd been adopted by a woman who didn't like her at all. That mother said terrible things, was cold and cruel, and often threatened to get rid of "the ugly, stupid little girl."

All that little baby knew was that she must be very unlovable indeed, having been rejected and emotionally abandoned by all of the women who had been "mother" to her.

That little girl was — and is — still a part of me. She was my first experience of this life. She's part of my past, and that will never change.

But what I *could* change was my response to what happened to her — to me. I had already done such a lot to heal. I had come such a long way. I didn't know if I would ever see the last of those wounds but I did know that the healing had always been ongoing.

This was just another step in the process. During my "on again" periods when I was smoking occasionally, I wasted tons of time and energy stressing about it, feeling ashamed, "Should I or shouldn't I?" Tormented by guilt, the negative self-talk that went with it was terrible. "I'm such an idiot! How can I be so stupid? I'm such a terrible person!" If someone had actually said those words to me, I would have called such behaviour abusive. It wasn't okay for my mother or others to do it, yet I was beating myself up. I might as well have applied those words with a baseball bat because they were at least as damaging and hurt far longer than that would have done.

How I longed to return to the days when smoking disgusted me and I hadn't wanted anything to do with it. The whole issue was doing my head in. I understood that by simply stopping smoking, I was not addressing the reason for the self-destructive desire to do it. I had to focus on resolving the problem and healing the cause of the addiction.

A life-changing thought occurred to me. I did not cause this addiction or this self-destructive streak. I was responsible for healing it, but I did not create it. And if I did not create it, then I had no reason to feel "bad" about it. I hadn't done anything "wrong" and therefore, had no reason to feel guilt.

The addiction came from deep wounds that were inflicted on me when I was a child and could not defend or protect myself. I had been immersed in a sea of shaming, destructive insults. I was belittled, shamed and ridiculed. I felt completely worthless. I could not be held responsible for the resulting damage.

Understanding this made all the difference in my ability to let go of the guilt associated with smoking so that I could better use that energy to focus on ways to heal the reasons for it. I realised that on top of the insults and abuse that had created this issue in me, any further self-hatred, self-recrimination and criticism were only adding to the negativity and perpetuating the self-defeating cycle that had driven me to take up smoking in recent years.

It is not enough to cut off a weed at ground level. You've got to yank it out by its roots.

So as I had done in various ways in the preceding 30 years or so, I tackled those wounds once again. This time, it was by writing the words "self-love" and "self-acceptance" on a piece of paper and putting it on the jug. Over the next several days, I drank plenty of water from that jug and I noticed that my craving for cigarettes subsided. Don't get me wrong; I still had my moments, especially when I was in the company of smokers. But honestly, it did get much easier and it happened fairly quickly, too.

In fact, within a week or two, there were times I felt disgusted by the thought of smoking, and if I attempted to have a cigarette when I was with a smoker, it made me sick. Now this was progress! I was delighted, to say the very least. I still had the odd craving, so I continued to drink from the jug. I left "self-love" and "self-acceptance" on it for some time, even after I had beaten the desire to smoke. Now, I am completely and utterly repulsed by the notion, and I feel sickened by the smell when I pass someone who is smoking. There is not a chance in hell that I will ever put another cigarette to my lips. The very idea of deliberately poisoning my precious body makes my skin crawl. Thank heaven.

In the few years just prior to this period, another problem had slid quietly into my life. My weight was at a place I did not appreciate. I had always been very underweight, but for some reason, it had suddenly begun to creep up a little at a time. For my age and height, I was still in the "normal, healthy range" (although nearing the top end of it). I was not overweight, but I felt like I was living in someone else's body and I was most uncomfortable about it, to say the least. I wanted my super thin body back, please.

To that end, I'd been paying more attention to what I ate and was weighing myself, worrying about calories and fat and what the scale said each morning. This had been going on for some time. Occasionally, I had the discipline to work at it and lose a little weight, then I'd get busy or depressed or both, and quit bothering. The numbers would sneak up once again.

Then one day, I noticed I hadn't been caring about my weight for weeks. I found myself not minding the extra bits of squishy around the middle. I wasn't worried about being near the top end of the "normal, healthy range" anymore. I loved and accepted my body as it was. I felt grateful for all the parts of it that worked, and for all the things it allowed me to do. I caught myself smiling at it, even giving it hugs, telling it how much I appreciated it.

This was all pretty weird for me — but it felt good. So I kept doing it. And after a few weeks, I realised what had happened. It had to have been because of putting "self-love" and "self-acceptance" on the jug of water. There was no other explanation. After years of stressing about my weight and hating how I looked, suddenly, quietly and almost magically, I was loving my body? I was accepting it as it was? That was no coincidence. I hadn't even thought about the issue of weight when I stuck those words on that jug. I was thinking only about trying to remove my self-destructive tendencies, especially with regard to smoking.

This was astonishing. With each of these experiments, I'd got a completely unexpected result. I was convinced it worked. Excited by this discovery, I began to suggest this to other people who were dealing with various emotional and physical issues. They tried it and soon were telling me that it seemed to be working for them, too.

I began to contemplate Dr. Emoto's work more seriously, having seen how profoundly the various energies of certain thoughts had affected the water. I thought about a couple of photos of ice crystals I'd seen in one of his books, the first being a disturbing image that looked like a distorted, anguished face. It had come from the lake at Fujiwara Dam in Japan.

The Reverend Kato Hoki, chief priest of the Jyuhouin Temple, sat facing the lake and prayed for one hour, after which another water sample was taken and frozen. This time, the ice produced clear, bright, stunning and detailed snowflake-like crystals. I read about Tokyo's tap water, which refused to produce ice crystals until 500 people transmitted the words "Chi, Soul and Spirit" to it.

And that's when it hit me. Just like the earth, we're approximately 70% water. I knew this already, but I hadn't considered the significance of this fact in terms of the energy in our environments. We must be absorbing every bit of it all the time! No wonder I always said I was so sensitive to the energy around me. For years, I'd told people that I could walk past someone who'd had a bad day and feel as though I'd been slammed with a bag of bricks. It was physically painful for me to be in certain situations, such as filthy, cluttered homes or buildings, or if I had to be with people whose energy was really negative.

I thought it was just due to the super-sensitivity that also made me a good psychic and medium, as this is quite usual in people with these abilities. But I reckon it was made worse by the fact that my poor body was taking the hit of negative energy, in large part because of the water content in its cells. It wasn't just a psychic or emotional response I felt in my body. It was a full-on physical response that was actually happening. I'm sure it happens to everyone but perhaps some of us are more aware of it than others, and that awareness is dependent upon the level of sensitivity to energy.

I couldn't help thinking about how much negative energy I'd absorbed or endured throughout my life, and I confess I had a moment (or two) of panic considering how much damage had been done to my poor body for all those decades, even going back to the moment of my conception. As a homeopath, I knew that experiences in the womb were often relevant to a patient's health issues. I had always understood this on an energetic level. But suddenly, I saw it in a whole new way. The tiny cluster of cells that makes up an embryo is 95% water. In babies and small children, it's about 80%. No wonder they're so sensitive to what's going on around them.

On realising this, I had an overwhelming need to protect myself from ever being subjected to any more negativity — and I hadn't even discovered one of the most sinister pieces of this puzzle yet. It lurks in places we wouldn't consider, some of which are hiding in plain sight. They're so common, such an enormous part of our everyday lives, that we'd never imagine the dangers to which we're exposed almost all the time.

Chapter Twenty-One

In Dr. Emoto's best-selling book, *The Hidden Messages in Water,* he raises an issue I'd heard in passing from time to time but had always ignored. With repeated testing giving consistent results, Dr. Emoto found that distilled water shown the words "love and gratitude" always produced beautiful ice crystals — but not when it had been left near computers, televisions, or mobile phones. The photographs of these crystals are honestly frightening. They look chaotic, dark, and splattered, just like the crystals formed from water exposed to heavy metal music or to words of anger or hatred. The crystal from water heated in a microwave even looked almost exactly like the one produced when water was shown the word "Satan."

In previous years, I'd occasionally heard about the harmful effects of electromagnetic waves but had never bothered to look into it. I figured, like so many other scary news flashes, it was probably just a lot of neurotic babbling with little or no validity. I couldn't have been more wrong.

When I saw Dr. Emoto's eerie photos of what electromagnetic waves do to water, a frightening thought hit me. It was as though someone had kicked me hard in the stomach when I realised that, being 70% water, we must be profoundly affected by the electromagnetic waves we're subjected to every day.

I looked around my flat and saw electricity and electronics everywhere — a small television, DVD player, CD player, lamps, fridge, cooker, toaster oven. The list went on. I grabbed my laptop, went online, and started digging into the effects of these invisible waves on the human body. It felt like stepping into a minefield. With one explosive bit of information after another, the more I found, the more I wished I could turn back time and un-know everything I was learning. To be honest, turning back time would have been easier than fixing or escaping the problem.

An electromagnetic field (EMF) is a field of energy created by electrically charged objects. Our homes, offices, cars, and lives are full of them. Wherever there's anything that uses electricity, there's an EMF. We can't escape them; there are live wires running behind the walls of every building in modern society. Overhead lights, electric toothbrushes, hair dryers, gadgets of all shapes and sizes, electric blankets, waterbed heaters, microwave ovens, mobile and portable phones, printers, scanners, X-rays, radio waves — the list goes on. Outside there are mobile phone towers, transformers, high-voltage power lines, electrical substations. If it needs electricity to operate, it's creating an EMF.

Exposure to EMFs is nothing new, as they're created naturally all over the world. But over the last century, our exposure has increased dramatically due to our heavy use of electricity and ongoing technological advances.

Over the years, EMFs have been blamed for a long list of ailments: non-specific aches and pains, digestive problems, sleep disturbances, exhaustion, depression, infertility, headaches, leukemia, immune system problems, hyperactivity, even cancer — just to name a few. There's been an enormous amount of research on this controversial topic. Countless studies claim EMFs do affect our health, but the World Health Organization (WHO) still says there's no clear link, adding that "some gaps in knowledge about biological effects exist and need further research."

So whom should we believe? Can thousands of studies and articles really all be wrong? And if there's no clear link between EMFs and our health, why does the WHO say on its website, "Fields of different frequencies interact with the body in different ways"? If there's an interaction between an EMF and the body, doesn't that at least suggest the possibility of an adverse effect?

Geobiology is the science of location and its impact on health, since there are so many environmental factors that can affect us. Former London Metropolitan Police Officer Roy Riggs is a geobiologist and professional dowser in the UK, and he's considered an expert in his field. Using scientific testing equipment, he measures the strength of EMFs for his clients. On the Body Ecology website, Riggs says, "When you are outside, your body comes into resonance with the earth's natural voltage. When you walk into your house, your body is actually the most conductive thing in your house, which means the EMFs are attracted right to you...and your voltage shoots up."

These words hit me like I'd slammed into a brick wall. First, I thought about the fact that we resonate with the earth's natural voltage. Of course we do. Why hadn't I noticed this before? We aren't just human beings, we are "of nature." We are one of the organisms that needs the earth to survive because we are part of it. And not only are we 70% water, so is the earth. Coincidence? I don't think so. There's a natural relationship there, a connection that can't be denied, as though we are tiny mini-earths. Of course we attune ourselves to the earth; we're just as much a part of it as every other animal or plant that survives on it and because of it.

As for being "the most conductive thing in your house," well, of course we are. Nothing else in our homes is 70% water, and isn't that just about the perfect conductor for electricity?

As I kept researching this worrying topic, I discovered that laptop computers are thought to be especially bad for EMFs. They should never be used directly on your lap, nor while plugged in and charging, because the transformer is especially dangerous. Horrified, I thought back over the previous 12 years or so — much of which I'd spent with my laptop on my lap or very close to me. I used it 14–18 hours a day on average, and when I wasn't actually using it, the laptop was usually at my feet or even on or under my bed while I slept, with the transformer (the most dangerous bit) plugged in and often just inches, or maybe a foot or two, from some part of my body.

When I looked at the long list of symptoms that some say may be caused by EMF exposure, I saw myself all over it. I thought back to the many times I'd tried a remedy or some other form of healing that seemed to work for a little while, and then stopped. Could it be that I might have had better results if I hadn't been constantly bombarded by EMFs? Knowing how terribly sensitive I am to the energies around me, it made perfect sense that I'd be affected by something like this. If I can't even cope with being in a very cluttered, untidy environment because it feels like a physical assault on my body, how could I cope with this?

Continuing my investigation, I stumbled upon an interesting bit of information: negative ions can reduce or even eliminate the effects of EMFs. Ions are molecules that have either gained or lost an electrical charge. Simply put, positively charged particles float in the air and attract mold, allergens, bacteria, dust, and so on. Negative ions are attracted to them and essentially weigh them down so they fall, making them less easily inhaled or ingested — and therefore the air we breathe is cleaner. Falling or moving water, like a waterfall, rainfall, or water fountain, generates lots of negative ions, which cleans the air and noticeably improves the environment. This is why people often report feeling relaxed, yet invigorated, exhilarated, and alert after it rains, or when they're by the sea.

Turning on the cold water in your shower or bath and letting it run for a few minutes is a natural ionizer for your home, as is burning pure beeswax or using indoor fountains. Plants are another great air cleaner, especially those with sharp, pointy leaves like pines and ferns, or those with a large leaf surface area. According to Wolverton Environmental Services, Inc., using their leaves, plants pull air down into their roots, giving them oxygen along with many airborne contaminants and organic chemicals. Microbes that live around the roots break down and convert many of these chemicals into food and energy, both for the plant and for themselves.

Another natural ionizer is the salt rock lamp, which you can get in all sorts of sizes, shapes and styles. Coincidentally — and knowing they're good air cleaners — shortly after moving into my flat I'd purchased several small, inexpensive ones from a website. I wanted to create the healthiest and most positive environment possible, not only for my patients and clients, but also for myself. I'd arrived back in Canada feeling completely broken and lost. I needed all the help I could get if I was going to put myself back together again, and I knew I was especially vulnerable to serious illness because of the intense emotional stress and depression I was feeling.

Reading about the potential EMF harm from cordless phones, computers, printers, wi-fi and so on made me want to get away from my laptop fast and start making some changes. At the time, I'd been keeping it plugged in at my feet where I usually sat in the sitting room — so whether I was working, reading or watching a bit of telly, that transformer was right there, spewing powerful electromagnetic waves at me during most of my waking hours.

Immediately, I set to work figuring out what I could do to lessen the EMF issue in my flat. The second bedroom was set up as an office, but for some reason, I didn't like being in it. There was a new desktop computer in there, too, as my laptop was well past its prime and should have been rocking on the porch of the nursing home for computers. But no matter what little things I changed, rearranged or reorganised, I just couldn't get myself to like being in that room.

Still, I was determined to sort things out and make friends with the office so I could stop using my laptop so much, or at least use it at my desk and have a bit more distance from it.

All of my electronic gadgetry was in the office — the wi-fi equipment, my desktop computer, external hard drive for back-up, my wireless printer/scanner/copier, my digital piano and electronic bits for recording. It was a veritable hotbed of EMFs in that little room. First, I needed to rearrange the furniture to make it feel better for me — no easy feat as there was a lot of it in a small space. There were so many cables from several bits of equipment and lamps, too many things plugged in, and too many extension cords. It was a huge electrical cabling nightmare.

In an effort to minimise the EMF concern, I had to work out which things could be shut off at the source of electricity and which needed to stay on — and with only a few electrical outlets and a ton of things to plug in, this was quite a challenge. It just about did my head in, but thankfully, I had some multi-plug power strips to use, and as a bonus, each of them could be turned off.

I persevered. After spending several hours rearranging and reorganising everything in my office, I'd managed to get the wi-fi components as far away from my desk chair as possible, along with some of the other major EMF offenders. I had a good-sized salt rock lamp on my desk, right next to my computer. Somehow, I even managed to get rid of what felt like miles of excess extension cords. My laptop was moved to a far corner of the office, with the transformer in the closet along with my wireless printer. That would now be plugged into an outlet that was turned off when not in use, and I had similarly sorted out all the other electronic components of the office.

It had been a logistical nightmare, but I'd done it. My office feels so much better now; it's inviting and feels much more positive — something others have noticed too. Whether or not it's because I've reduced the EMFs significantly, I will never know. I just know that I love it and I look forward to spending time in my office, whereas before making these changes, I wouldn't go in unless I had no choice.

169

This wasn't the first "environmental cleanse" I'd done as I worked to create a new and healthier life for myself in Canada. I had done something far more drastic than this — something that forced me to make some of the most difficult decisions I'd ever made in my life.

Chapter Twenty-Two

Science tells us that everything is made up of energy. In his book *A Happy Pocket Full of Money*, David Cameron Gikandi explains, "[Energy] is the building block of all matter. The same energy that composes your flesh is the same one that composes the bricks of your house and the trees outside. It is all the same."

Further, Einstein said that energy can be neither created nor destroyed.

Therefore, everything that exists holds energy, always.

As a highly sensitive individual, I've always been profoundly impacted by the energy around me. Both a blessing and a curse, as I mentioned earlier, this has made me a very perceptive psychic and medium, but it has also been the source of a lot of illness, anxiety, and emotional upset.

Once it became clear that I had no sensible choice but to return to Canada, I had to begin the task of deciding what to take with me. Having made one international move already, I knew well the expense involved in shipping furniture and other belongings to another country. I had to take a good, hard look at what I could take and what I would need to leave behind.

Because of other circumstances in the past, I had already lost many personal items — including my home and almost everything I owned in Canada — due to my move to England. I had faced the lesson of "letting go" on numerous occasions, and although I understood that I shouldn't cry over anything that couldn't cry over me, I loved the beautiful antiques I had collected and many gifts and special little bits and pieces of my life that I had accumulated over the years.

Part of the problem for me was that, even worse than losing material possessions, I was losing my entire life in England — everything familiar about my day-to-day existence, the people I saw regularly, my beloved English "family." Not knowing what lay ahead, I had to face the fact that once I left, I might never see any of them or set foot on English soil again.

Those roots that I'd worked so hard to plant were mighty deep, and I was being forced to rip them out — all of them, all at once. Leaving behind even my beautiful furniture and favourite personal items added insult to injury. But it was the sensible thing to do under the circumstances.

As I considered which items I could take and which I would have to leave behind, I began to think about the energy each one held. Many carried the bittersweet energy of a failed marriage, leaving me conflicted about whether to keep them — wanting to remember the good, yet reminded of the pain.

It was then that I thought about feng shui. Developed thousands of years ago, it's the Chinese art of practical ecology, involving the positioning, colour, and type of objects, furnishings — virtually everything — to improve the flow of energy, or "Qi" (pronounced "chee"), in homes, offices, and other spaces. According to feng shui, the earth has "veins" of energy coursing through it and holding it together. These veins act as a grid from which all life derives its power, or Qi. This energy — this life force — is everywhere, and it can move freely or become stagnant and blocked. If practiced properly, it is said to improve and maintain health, wealth, business, relationships — essentially all areas of life. It's extremely complex, but fascinating.

I had heard bits and pieces about feng shui over the years and had always intended to study it. Because it involves the participation of all members of a household in order to do it properly, it had never seemed feasible in the past. But as I was starting fresh in a new flat, with a blank canvas in terms of deciding what to take, and as the only one responsible for the move, it seemed like the perfect time to give it a try.

I began researching feng shui online and bought a couple of books on the subject. Over and over, I read stories of people who used to think it was a load of rubbish, or who had reluctantly given it a grumpy and begrudging try after being pressured by a spouse, only to find amazing, positive results very quickly. I was giving up so much for this move; I had to make sure it was worthwhile. It was imperative that I should do everything I could to turn my life around, to improve my health, and to use every tool available to me, so that this overwhelming move would ultimately become a positive experience — one that I would not regret.

I began communicating with Dawn Hankins, a feng shui expert in Calgary, and arranged to have her meet me at my flat a couple of nights after my arrival. As a teacher of feng shui at Mount Royal University, and host of her own feng shui television show, I figured I was in good hands.

During my last months in England, Dawn and I exchanged numerous emails as I sought her guidance to make my choices. Some of them were relatively simple; others were quite difficult. But having made the commitment to practice the principles of feng shui, there was no point in picking and choosing the ones I liked and ignoring the ones I didn't. If not following the rules was potentially going to diminish or eliminate any benefits I might gain, then I was wasting my time. The way I saw it, it's like you can't be "sort of pregnant." Either you are or you aren't. You either do it or you don't. It had to be all or nothing if I was going to give it a fair chance to prove that it worked—or didn't.

One of the first things I learned was that I had to absolutely love or absolutely need every single item in my home, no matter how small or seemingly inconsequential. This sounds easy enough, but it becomes difficult in certain circumstances. For example, what do you do with gifts or mementos that you don't absolutely love or need, but were given to you by special people, and you worry about offending them by not keeping the items? Or you enjoy the memory but not the object? Or what if you absolutely love objects that hold a load of sentimental value, but there is an element of sadness, loss, or grief?

The short answer: These items have to go. The more you follow feng shui principles, the more positive the energy flow, and the better your chances of obtaining the desired results.

There were some very emotional stumbling blocks over items connected to the marriage I mentioned above — many much-loved mementos and gifts. Although they made me smile as I remembered happier days a lifetime ago, they also brought tears of heartache and sadness. For that reason, I had to part with them. Only the ones that left me smiling were okay to keep. To be honest, there weren't many on that list.

Having made the brutal decision to leave almost all of my beautiful antiques behind to cut the shipping cost as much as possible, it became easier to let go of the smaller bits of my life. As I made my way through each item, I found myself letting go of far more than I kept. I needed to keep expenses down, but I was determined to hang onto my very most favourite and necessary belongings.

Until I came to a few in particular. I knew, before even asking Dawn, that she would tell me they had to go. I didn't want to know. I tried to tell myself that it was only a few, just these five little bits, and perhaps they would not matter very much, as I was going above and beyond what was necessary in so many other ways.

But I was kidding myself, and I knew it.

Although I'd had several cats in my life, I had the ashes of only one of them. She'd had an especially lovely personality, and I'd had her longer than any other pet — fifteen years.

There was a tiny eagle "ornament" that contained a small amount of my father's ashes, and a little box with a lock of his silky soft grey hair that I'd collected after his death. These, I could not keep, so I put them aside and wound up giving them to one of my daughters in Calgary.

For all the difficulties I experienced growing up under the black cloud of my father's alcoholism, eventually I remembered that, amidst my mother's constant criticism and insults, my dad used to tell me that I was beautiful, that I was smart, that I could be anything I wanted to be. He said he loved me. He didn't say such things very often, but at least he said them. For many years, they remained buried under the nastiness my mother had heaped on top of me.

When those special memories of my father surfaced during a load of healing work in my early 30s, I made my peace with him, realizing that I loved him. It was his alcoholism I'd hated while growing up, but I forgave him, finally understanding that he had done his best. There was healing on both sides, and during the remaining years of his life, my father and I had been extremely close. For that, I am truly grateful.

The last two items on my feng shui "hit list" were the most difficult of all, and I'm sure I will never find words to adequately convey the depth of my feelings about them, or about the relationship I had with my beloved little Bob. Thirteen years old when he died, he was one of my snakes, my buddy, my dopey little pal who was loaded with personality and really quite funny. An eight-foot rat snake, he had made the big move to England with me all those years ago.

Snakes are extremely sensitive animals and bond very closely with their owners. Bob and I were particularly close. He would go off his food when I was experiencing some emotional turmoil or other; he was always aware if things weren't right with me, and his behaviour changed accordingly. If I was happy, Bob was happy. If I was not, neither was he.

If you're like most people, you may be surprised to learn that snakes are very gentle and timid, and will go out of their way not to bite anyone. They are usually very much misunderstood, which I suppose is why I had such an affinity for them — for that has been my experience of life, too. Bob was very curious for a snake, and he loved people, although he approached them cautiously from the safety of my shoulders or peeking out from my hair. I absolutely adored my little Bob, like no other cat, dog, or snake I'd ever owned.

Although he was getting on for a rat snake, he could have had a few more years, but he developed a painful tumour in his tummy and had to be put down a year and a half before my move back to Canada. Several months before he died, Bob had managed to shed in one perfect piece, from his nose and eye caps all the way down to the tip of his tail. This was extremely rare, as the skin is so delicate that it normally tears into at least a few pieces. I had kept this skin; there was nothing more important to me among my possessions. I had no intention of parting with it, until Dawn told me that it was forbidden in feng shui practice.

I'd made the commitment to practice feng shui. I had to see it through; I had to see if it would help me to move on in my life, to move forward and reach a point of healing, success, and happiness. That meant I had no choice. Amidst buckets of tears, I let go of Bob's skin.

No doubt you can guess the fifth item — Bob's ashes. I saved those for a special goodbye in Calgary. A few weeks after my arrival, I took them to Carburn Park. When my children were young, we went there regularly for walks, as it was near our home. Every time we passed one particularly beautiful big tree beside the Bow River, I would always have a different story for my children about Mrs. Bunny and her babies who lived under it.

I sat under that tree on the bank of the river that crisp winter morning, clutching the small container of Bob's ashes close to my heart. Amidst a flood of tears, he and I had a quiet little heart-to-heart. It was almost as emotional as the one we'd had in the hours before we said goodbye at the veterinary clinic, except that on that very painful day, he had been wrapped tightly around my shoulders, with his little face buried in the side of my neck. Bless him; it was as though he was comforting me that day, rather than fearing his own terrible death (snakes must be injected directly in the heart; you cannot see their veins...).

This time, all I had of him was a little plastic jar full of powder. I took my time by the river, watching the sun sparkling on the water and remembering my little pal. How sweet and funny he was! How much joy he had brought to my life! I'd been more blessed by our many years together than I could have ever imagined. I'd loved and lost several pets since I was a child, but this loss was especially terrible. I did not think I would ever have another pet after this.

Finally, I was ready. I knew that after this day, I would never see any physical trace of my precious little Bob again. It would be almost as though he had never existed. But I knew I would still feel his sweet and gentle spirit and his loving hugs every time I thought about him.

Two days after arriving in Calgary, it was most interesting to meet with Dawn and some of her students. I learned all the things I needed to do in order to sort out my flat, the point of which was to sort out my health, career, and all other aspects of my new life. Once she understood my situation and problems, as well as what I hoped to achieve, she used feng shui principles to help me with such decisions as the placement of furnishings, and which room was best for my office, based on the type of work I wanted to attract. I was advised about various "cures" for energy flow problems such as "arguing doors." I was told where to hang crystals or wind chimes, where to put mirrors, which rooms required the addition of specific colours, or where and how to add the elements of wood, water, fire, metal, and wind to create balance.

I was told where to put information or objects related to travel if I wanted to attract more of it into my life. I learned how to decorate my bedroom to attract balanced and harmonious loving relationships (of all kinds). I had to be sure no electrical wires were touching any part of my bed, and it was best not to have a television, CD player, or any other electronic devices in my room.

I learned what to do in my office to create the best flow of creative energy. I learned the importance of having a water feature, or a symbol that represented water, near my door. The more I learned, the more fascinated I was. I had quite a list of requirements to fulfill, but it was exciting and interesting; I enjoyed setting to work, shopping for the little bits and pieces I needed, such as red thread or ribbon, the wind chimes, mirrors, and so on. I did as much as I could while waiting for my belongings to arrive from England.

Interestingly, once they had been delivered and I'd unpacked and worked my way through the feng shui list of things to do, people who came round would comment on how calm and serene my flat was. It wasn't just people who knew I'd used feng shui either. For example, a woman brought her 12-year-old son to me for homeopathy treatment. I was shocked when about ten minutes into our appointment, he commented on the peaceful "energy" in my flat and said he felt unusually relaxed. His mother piped up, agreeing that it was very tranquil and saying that, as her son was ordinarily very wound up and restless, it was a huge surprise to see him so calm and settled.

If I'm honest, I would have to say I did not expect any particular results when I used feng shui on my flat. I suppose I was hopeful, but did I really think it was going to improve my sleep or my health? Probably not. Did I really believe it would help my career? I was dubious, at best. And if it was going to produce these miracles, I figured it would take some time. It was nice to think about the possibilities, but I wasn't holding my breath. I just did what I had been taught to do and got on with rebuilding my life.

Despite the depression and emotional distress over my move to Canada, over the several weeks it took to sort out my flat and look after the business end of creating a new life, I was surprised to discover that I'd been sleeping better and longer than I'd done in more than 30 years. It was a few weeks before I noticed that I hadn't been dragging my sorry behind through my days, and also, that my headaches had vanished. This was especially intriguing, as I'd been plagued with such bad ones almost every day for decades, and they were always particularly nasty in Calgary because of the erratic weather and high altitude.

For two months I tore up the city, running here and there to get things done, and when I was back home in my flat, I kept rearranging this and that, or running out to get another "organizer" from Walmart and dashing back to put some order to another closet or cupboard. Physically, I was holding up remarkably well in terms of joint pain, heart trouble, kidney issues—the usual assortment of "stuff." They were not gone, but I had to admit that there had been some improvement.

Then, over a period of several weeks, my symptoms crept back. I didn't notice at first; it was so gradual. One day, I realised I was no longer sleeping as well or as long as I'd done in those first two months. My headaches had returned. I was exhausted again. My joints (particularly that miserable hip and my knees) were giving me as much grief as ever. Having followed every one of the feng shui principles I learned, and then seeing the dramatic improvements in my sleep and overall health, I was terribly disappointed and confused. It was like having that big dangling carrot yanked away. After years of striving to get it, I'd had it ever so briefly—and now it was gone.

But why? How could this happen? I hadn't changed anything in my flat since I finished doing everything the feng shui consultant had advised me to do. I was still minding all the rules. What was different?

The answer smacked me right between the eyes.

Chapter Twenty-Three

I had hit rock bottom. For decades, I'd tried anything and everything I could think of that might help me. Feng shui had felt like at least a partial answer — a little flicker of hope. For two months after beginning to use it, I'd actually noticed improvements in my sleep and my health. But then it all vanished. Discouraged and completely disheartened, I lost all hope. And then I got angry. As you know, it was that anger that finally spilled over one day and became the determination to figure out how to heal myself.

It was fairly early in my self-healing investigations that I stumbled across some very unsettling information about EMFs. More specifically, I learned how harmful it can be to use a laptop — especially one that's plugged in and charging while being used, and especially when it's not on a desk or paired with a separate keyboard and mouse. In other words, I was doing everything wrong. No wonder I was miserable, sleeping poorly, and feeling so unwell.

But then, a question popped up: if my laptop was the problem, why had there been such a big improvement in my health for a couple of months after moving here — particularly when I was in

180

such a state of emotional turmoil? You'd think that would have made me worse, not better.

And suddenly, I put two and two together. During my first two months back in Calgary, I'd barely touched my laptop. I was far too busy organising my new life to do any writing or work, and I didn't even have internet for a while. I had no time or interest for anything computer-related anyway as I tried to adjust to life in Canada. And when I did finally have a little time for email or Facebook, I was usually too emotionally drained, homesick or just plain exhausted to be very communicative.

It was only once I'd finished sorting out my flat and the business end of my move that I got back to building a new website, designing advertising, writing and recording more meditation CDs, and slipping back into a more normal life. That meant my laptop usage went right back up to an average of 14–16 hours a day. It took a couple of months, but gradually I slid right back into my old pattern of poor sleep and declining health.

Without even meaning to, I'd just completed two experiments. I hadn't expected any results from feng shui and, truth be told, I hadn't held out much hope either. But then the light went on after a few weeks of improvement — some of my biggest complaints had quietly disappeared. Apparently, feng shui works.

It also seemed clear that there was truth to the EMF issue. I'd known nothing about it during those first months — certainly not about the dangers of laptops — yet when I resumed using mine, my symptoms returned. Maybe the harmful effects of electromagnetic waves are more obvious to those of us who are especially sensitive to our environment — whether that's allergies, energies, or weather changes. But that doesn't mean it isn't affecting people who don't consciously notice the more subtle influences around them. After all, they're 70% water, just like me. Their bodies are made up of charged particles, just like mine.

Even if we aren't aware of them, electric and magnetic fields still induce voltages and currents in the body. We can't help but be affected by the overwhelming amount of artificially generated electromagnetic waves in our technologically overloaded society. The body is designed to protect and heal itself, and it can do so when it gets a break from offending or toxic substances and environments. But when there's no relief from ongoing assaults, the body becomes stressed. That leads to a wide range of symptoms and degenerative diseases as we slip into long-term protection — the "fight or flight" mode.

When it comes to EMFs, there's a lot we can do to reduce any long-term effects. Buying ionisers, salt rock lamps, or water fountains and placing them near electronics is a good start. Keeping windows open when weather permits can also help cut EMFs in your home or office. Limiting your exposure to mobiles, laptops, and other portable devices — or to electronics in general — will make a huge difference. If you must keep a mobile or pager handy, try leaving it nearby rather than right next to your body.

Unplug as many electrical items as you can when they are not in use. If you must have a portable phone, don't leave it next to your bed or furniture where you spend long periods of time. Whether or not you believe you are being affected by EMFs, it can't hurt and it might help to reduce your exposure to them, thereby lessening the potential for any health problems. It will improve the flow of Qi in your home, too, which will also affect the flow of Qi in your body.

According to Chinese medicine, Qi flows along 12 meridians that run through the body, much like the "veins of energy" that are said to course through the earth in a sort of grid. When the flow of Qi in the body becomes blocked or is too strong or too weak, imbalances occur and we see symptoms. Acupuncture works by removing blockages and restoring balance in the flow of Qi.

Early in my self-healing project, I was thinking about my acupuncture days many years earlier. It occurred to me that apart from the scarring on my heart, there was no structural damage to my kidneys or other parts of my body that had been contributing to my ill health. If they could have been physically examined, they would appear to be just fine. According to the principles of Chinese medicine, the problem was not of a physical nature; it was entirely related to energy weakness. In later chapters, you will see how I applied this principle to my self-healing project, as I sought to restore balance in my body and in my life.

Everything in nature requires balance to function effectively. Because everything is in motion, all processes are cyclical. There is always change, an ebb and flow. There is heat and there is cold, light and dark, night and day. We cannot have one without the other. It is the same with emotions; love and hate are just two ends of the same spectrum with "like" somewhere in the middle. If you look at the yin/yang symbol with its equal parts of white and black, you will see that each has a little dot of the opposite colour inside it. This is because each contains the seed of the other, just as day gradually becomes night, and then night gradually becomes day.

Yin is cold, heavy, dark, unmoving, wet, solid and contraction. Yang is hot, light, movement, dry, and expansion. Yin is quiet and static; Yang is dynamic and active. We need both in equal measure in the environment, in our homes, in our bodies, and in our lives.

For example, think about what life would be like if you worked 18 hours every day of the week. You never take a day off. You sleep a few hours, grab a fast meal when you can and spend the rest of your waking hours at work. Can you imagine how quickly this would take a toll on your health and your happiness?

Likewise, if all you ever did was sit and stare at a computer and play on the internet or watch the telly, and you did not look after your responsibilities or your household obligations, if you did not bother to go to work, if you did not take care of laundry, bill-paying, socialising or proper meals, what sort of life would that be? If working 18 hours a day is unhealthy, it does not mean that playing 18 hours a day is any better. Simply put, 180 degrees from sick is still sick. We need balance. A time to work, a time to rest, a time to play and take care of ourselves. All are required in the pursuit of good health.

All foods are considered to be either yin or yang, and therefore, a healthy diet will require a balance of both. However, if you have either a deficiency or an excess of yin or yang in your body, your food choices will contribute to your illness or your healing. We should also eat yang foods in the morning when our bodies and the world are still yin, and yin foods during the day when our bodies and the world are yang. Warming foods when it is cooler, cooling foods when it is warmer. This is how we achieve balance.

Although we cannot see the meridians in the body, nor can we see the energy grid in the earth, it is apparent that the balance of yin and yang energies in our lives and in our bodies is imperative for our wellbeing. Both Chinese medicine and feng shui have withstood the tests of time, as each one is still going strong after a few thousand years.

Homeopathy is similar to acupuncture, in that it seeks to restore homeostatis, which is the ability of an organism to regulate its internal environment, for example its temperature. More simply put, it is about maintaining balance. Homeopathic philosophy teaches us that we are born with various weaknesses and susceptibilities that have been handed down from previous generations. This is referring to weaknesses on an energetic level, not a physical or genetic level. In perfect health, we would function with complete freedom on all levels: mentally, emotionally and physically. The mental level is said to be the most important for human functioning, happiness and creativity, the emotional level a close second, and the physical being the third.

For example, imagine a person who has paranoid schizophrenia and who hears threatening, frightening voices in his head day and night, but has perfect physical health. No aches or pains, no illnesses, never gets sick. Is this person going to have any sense of freedom, creativity, or happiness? Hardly.

Imagine a woman who is quadriplegic, confined to a wheelchair and only able to move her head. She has no feeling or use of her body below her neck. But she paints with her mouth, she writes stories by dictation, she enjoys participating in family events, she "dances" with her husband, although she does it from her chair while he dances in front of her, holding her hands, or twirling her in her chair. Does this woman have a sense of freedom, creativity and happiness? Absolutely.

In Chinese medicine, the energy that drives us is called Qi, and in homeopathy, it is called the vital force. According to homeopathic philosophy, the body is capable of healing itself, and the vital force does so by creating symptoms in an effort to throw off "disease" (meaning any symptoms that interfere with our health, well-being and happiness) and reach a point of homeostasis. When we suppress symptoms, the vital force has to work harder to fight back and express what is out of balance, which further weakens it and creates worse or more serious symptoms.

For example, a child may have a bit of eczema. Nothing serious; just uncomfortable and itchy. But we give a steroid cream to suppress the symptom. After a time, the child begins to have allergies. These may become more serious; certainly they are more bothersome, with running and itching in the eyes and nose. It is definitely worse than a bit of eczema, for which we continue to pile on the steroid cream.

The allergies are a nuisance, so we begin giving antihistamines or possibly allergy shots. Some allergies may already be life-threatening, causing anaphylactic shock. But for the day-to-day, run-of-the-mill allergies, we continue to give drugs to eliminate symptoms, or to prevent them.

Before you know it, the child has asthma. Definitely a life-threatening, more serious problem than your average allergies. And then we're onto giving daily steroids preventatively, and there are the emergency inhalers for the flare-ups; we mustn't have any symptoms!

Or a patient has cancer. A big fat tumour sitting somewhere in the body and the surgeon goes in, cuts it out and says "Yay! It came out clean as a whistle! We got every bit of it!" Sure, get rid of the tumour, and call the patient cured.

This is the view of allopathic (conventional/traditional) medicine. You remove the symptoms and say you've cured the disease. In

185

homeopathy, we would rather cure the patient. This means removing the reason for the symptoms, thereby eliminating the need for them - a true cure. An example of this is when someone suppresses a load of anger or grief. It needs to be expressed but instead, the body (more accurately, the vital force) takes that negative energy and creates a tumour out of it. In a way, it's the vital force attempting to contain the negative energy and keep you safe. But of course, it is negative. It will only do you harm.

If you cut out the tumour but do not deal with the emotional issues that created it, your very unimpressed vital force says, "Hey! I needed that! Well, fine! I'll just grow another one over **here!**" And it finds somewhere else to set up a little tumour camp of rebellion.

If homeopathic philosophy states that symptoms are the vital force's efforts to heal us, then why do we not just automatically get well on our own, apart from those flus and broken bones I mentioned earlier? Well, the vital force is weakened by the energetic susceptibilities we inherit at birth. It is further weakened by the stresses in our lives, whether from emotional issues, trauma, shock, environmental factors, poor diet - there are loads of reasons why the vital force can't quite do it all on its own. It's like a crack in a dam. That tiny crack appears to be nothing all by itself. The dam still holds. But over time, the pressure builds, the crack grows, the weakness gets worse, the integrity goes and eventually, the dam bursts.

A weakened vital force will continue to try to correct itself. However, as we move through life and its many stressors, if we're not taking good care of ourselves, or if we suppress symptoms, the weakness only grows. In general, we have more symptoms, which makes us more stressed, which gives us more symptoms. And so on.

I used to worry about the damage I was doing to myself by suppressing the desire for beef before Simon suggested that I ought to eat it. I was well aware that I felt much better for having it, but struggled with the ethical issues around it, as I explained previously. Having discovered that it is medicinal for Type O individuals, with the high acid content of their bodies to digest meat, it made sense that I craved it when I had become so ill.

But what was up with the growing interest in chocolate? I'd never really had much of a sweet tooth, so why had I begun craving it from time to time, over the past couple of years? Aware of the damage caused by suppression of the desire, I was relieved to see that it was on the list of "allowed" foods on the Type O diet, so I indulged in small pieces of various chocolate bars from time to time. But it was not often, due to the sugar, fat and other ingredients that were entirely unnecessary and not particularly healthful, and it was just too sweet. Why would I crave chocolate bars when they're so bad for me, and when I couldn't cope with the sweetness?

It was only whilst I was doing research for this book that I stumbled upon some startling information that revealed possible answers to my questions.

Chapter Twenty-Four

I was happy to see that Type O is allowed to have chocolate, and whilst I was doing research for this book, I discovered an even happier surprise. Dark chocolate (with at least 70% content in bars) and cocoa have significant health benefits — and especially where the heart is concerned. Who'd have thought?!

In 2006, a team of Dutch researchers finished a 15-year study of 470 elderly men and concluded that "...the men who consumed the most cocoa-containing products...were half as likely to die from cardiovascular disease as those who consumed the least." (Buijsse B. Feskens EJM, Kof FJ, Kromhout D. Cocoa intake, blood pressure and cardiovascular mortality: the Zutphen Elderly Study. *Arch Intern Med* 2006; 166:411-7)

Dark chocolate and cocoa are loaded with flavanols, which are a key to heart health because of their ability to deactivate the unstable and dangerous free radicals in your bloodstream. Flavanols also help to stimulate the production of nitric oxide, which, as you may recall, our three Nobel prize winners discovered is responsible for relaxing arteries. This improves blood flow to every cell of the body, reducing blood pressure and helping in the treatment and prevention of numerous other problems.

Flavanols are also antioxidant powerhouses, which means, as you know from previous chapters, they help prevent cardiovascular disease, premature aging, and many degenerative diseases such as cancer. They can reduce cholesterol, and particularly the potential for damage caused by LDL. They have mild anti-clotting effects, improve blood flow, and may help with the prevention of atherosclerosis.

As if that isn't enough, dark chocolate and cocoa contain a variety of minerals, including a good portion of the daily requirement of copper, magnesium and potassium — and even some iron — in an average-sized bar. They also contain Phenylethylamine (PEA), which releases endorphins, "feel-good" chemicals in the brain. Interestingly, the brain produces PEA when people are falling in love. Eating some dark chocolate can give you a bit of that same yummy feeling.

The Aztecs and the Maya used to add a bit of chili to their cocoa drinks, so it is no surprise that we see this delicious combination becoming increasingly available in shops and restaurants in desserts and dark chocolate bars. Aside from being a real taste treat, the addition of chili has further health benefits. Chili peppers contain capsaicin, which research is now showing prevents fat cells from developing, thereby reducing both body fat, and the amount of fat that gets into the blood. Capsaicin has also been linked to killing certain cancer cells, and to boosting metabolism and burning more calories. Eating a bit of chili-infused dark chocolate every day - what a great way to drop a few pounds!

Having discovered the significant benefits to cardiovascular health, finally I understood why I was craving chocolate. The bars of milk chocolate that I had been having now and then were not particularly helpful but my vital force didn't send me a memo about the healthier dark stuff. All I knew was that I wanted chocolate, and as I thought dark chocolate was that horrible, bitter, unsweetened stuff that my mother used to use for baking, it would never have occurred to me to try it. I couldn't have been more wrong.

Thankfully, my research led me to try the chili-infused 70% dark chocolate bars, and oh, my goodness, what a yummy way to kill the craving and give my body the cardiovascular assistance it is requesting! In fact, without the milk and very little sugar, these bars packed a much bigger chocolate punch, so it didn't take much to satisfy me, and I didn't have to cope with awful sweetness.

As I have said in previous chapters in various ways, the body has intelligence. When we listen to its wisdom, we cannot go wrong. This is one of the fundamental principles of homeopathy, and my cravings for beef and chocolate, and the benefits that both could give me, seemed to substantiate it.

Around the globe, there is a great debate about homeopathic remedies being useless because it is believed that they are nothing more than water on a sugar pill. They are made from substances in nature that are diluted until there are no actual molecules of the original substance left, and therein lies the problem that many people have in understanding or accepting that there is any medicinal value in the remedies.

But there is science behind this very powerful method of healing, and much of it is science that we have already seen in previous chapters.

First, a bit of history. Samuel Hahnemann was a German doctor who lived in the 1700s. An exceptionally brilliant man, he was fluent in several languages by the age of 12. Fed up with the barbaric medical practices of that era, he turned to translating medical documents in order to support his family. Whilst translating a book (*A Treatise on Materia Medica*, by Dr William Cullen), he read that Peruvian Bark was used in the treatment of malaria, but that if it was given in overdose, it would **cause** symptoms of the disease instead.

His curious mind took him back more than 2,000 years to the words of Hippocrates, who was credited with the first writing of the

Law of Similars, "By similar things a disease is produced and through the application of the like is cured."

Aristotle, who lived from 384-322 BC, knew this principle, too, and wrote, "Often the simile acts upon the simile." Hahnemann summed up both of these statements by saying "Like cures like", or in the traditional Latin, he said, "Similia similibus curentur."

Quoted as saying he saw more people die from their treatments than from their diseases, which included bloodletting, leeching, and the use of terribly toxic substances, Hahnemann was eager to find a safer way to cure illness. Bravely, he did what homeopaths refer to as "the first proving of a remedy." That is to say, he took small doses of the Peruvian Bark until he began having symptoms, about which he wrote in great detail.

He continued testing, or "proving" numerous other substances, as did many other people who were intrigued and interested in finding a safer way to treat disease. Bless them, this had to have been most unpleasant, as they were offering to become violently ill, experience hallucinations, fears, pain — all sorts of nasty symptoms in the interests of discovering what the tested substances would cure.

Some of the information came from what was already known about the effects of poisons, chemicals and so on. As the number of provings grew, so did the detailed collection of mental, emotional and physical symptoms that were caused by these various substances. Before long, Hahnemann could see very separate and distinct pictures arising from each one, which allowed him to help increasing numbers of people.

As word about Hahnemann and his new medicine spread, Constantine Hering, a medical student and lover of the natural sciences, was hired to write a book disproving homeopathy but the more he learned about it, the more impressed he became — and the book was never published. Eventually, he and Hahnemann grew to be close friends, with Hering contributing to the development of Hahnemann's theories. As a pioneer of homeopathy in America who was responsible for spreading news of this powerful method of healing, Hering was the founder of the first school of homeopathy to be created anywhere in the world.

More than 200 years on, people all over the globe continue to do provings, adding to the wealth of information in the Materia Medica by creating new remedies. As the list grows, so does our ability to heal with homeopathy. I am reminded of a fascinating group "proving", of sorts, that was done at one of the homeopathy workshops I attended. Whilst out on a walk during the lunch break one day, one of the instructors had found a type of moss that had not yet been proven. When our class of approximately 35 people assembled for the afternoon session, he gave each of us a tiny bit of the moss to hold, directing us to sit quietly and make notes of anything that we experienced.

To be honest, I felt quite silly and expected absolutely nothing to happen. But I did as I was told, as did the rest of the group. Surprisingly, within minutes, I was aware of the sensation of pins and needles in my feet. Gradually, it moved up my calves to my knees and it was worse on the right than on the left. I recall feeling a sense of oppression in my chest, a sort of heaviness, and tightness. There was a bit of anxiety, some odd little pains in my stomach, and a feeling of sadness. I was overcome with the urge to cry for no apparent reason, but choked back the tears. There was more, and some of the symptoms were minor but noticeable, nonetheless.

Once we had finished writing our lists, the instructor has us go round the room and read what we had written. I was astonished to discover that collectively, we had all experienced the same symptoms in various combinations. Apparently, by bringing the moss into our own energy fields and focusing our attention on it, we were able to "tune in" and feel its effects on us.

Everything in nature is energy. Everything has its own particular vibrational frequency, which is why, for example, everyone has heard about glass shattering whilst an opera singer belts out a long, loud note.

To explain this phenomenon, we must look at a tuning fork,

which resonates at a specific pitch when struck against or with an object. It will produce a pure musical tone as it vibrates at a particular frequency. If you were to strike a second tuning fork of the same pitch, you might expect to hear two identical tones, just as you would if you recorded yourself singing, and then played it back whilst singing along. However, with two tuning forks of the same pitch, they resonate with one another, intensifying their vibrations and together producing one much louder tone, rather than two identical but discernible ones.

This is why we sometimes hear jokes or stories about an opera singer shattering glass. We know that all matter is made up moving molecules, with everything having its own particular vibrational frequency. And we know that sound waves have their own vibrational frequencies, too.

It should come as no surprise, then, that if there is an ongoing sound, for example the singing of a long note, if its vibrational frequency is the same as that of the glass, the glass will resonate with it and increase its frequency until it shatters. This is the Law of Similars in action. If we can find a substance in nature that has been known to produce the same symptoms as a patient already has, then that substance will bring about a cure.

At the risk of getting weighted down in details here, I must skip to the highlights, although this is a truly fascinating subject, all on its own.

Ultimately, Hahnemann began experimenting with diluting the substances, and pounding the vials hard (which he called "succussion") on his leather-bound Bible, which releases the energy from the substance into the water. The more diluted the physical substance, the more powerful its energy became.

If you think about Dr Emoto's brilliant experiments with water and the startling discoveries they revealed, homeopathy makes perfect sense. Knowing that everything in nature is made up of energy, which science has been proving for a very long time, and knowing that water "remembers" the energy in words, it is no surprise that it also retains the energy from the substances in nature that are used to create remedies.

I have often heard people say that you have to believe in homeopathy for it to work, but this is rubbish. I've seen it calm fussy babies, turn breech ones and prevent C-sections. I've seen it dramatically improve the mental and emotional functioning of patients with autism or Down's Syndrome. It rouses patients out of comas. It works on pets and little children for behavioural problems and all sorts of ailments. None of these patients would have any knowledge or understanding of having been given medicine, yet with the correct prescription, the results are astonishing.

Typically, only one dose is given and it is left for several weeks or months to do its work because it is not acting on a physical level. Rather, it has stimulated the vital force, given it a boost of energy that is similar to its own vibrational frequency, and allowing it that extra bit of strength it needed to throw off the symptoms and find its way to homeostasis.

We can see the Law of Similars attempting to help us find that point of balance when we are very cold. Many people run for a hot drink, thinking this will warm them up, when in fact, a cold drink will do it much quicker. Why? Because the vital force is always trying to keep us, or bring us back to, a position of homeostasis. If you get a fever, your body has ways to cool you. If you are cold, it shivers, creating muscle contractions that are designed to generate heat. The vital force knows the balance point between wet and dry, hot and cold, etc.

Therefore, if you have a hot drink, internally your vital force is thinking, "This is too hot! I need to cool down!" And it will make you feel colder. If you burn your fingers, you run them under cold water, which feels wonderful — until you take them out. Then they sting like mad.

Why? Because your vital force is aware of that excessive cold water. That's all it feels. So it effectively sends heat to warm it up, therefore making the burn hurt even more. If you put your fingers under water that is as hot as you can stand it for a few minutes, you will find quicker relief from the pain of the burn — and faster healing, too. Try it next time you burn yourself. I know it seems weird but it works. It is the Law of Similars; it always works, and it is the reason why homeopathy works, too.

Before I began homeopathy treatments, I was freezing all the time. On a summer's day, I could always be found indoors, wrapped in a sweater and buried under a quilt. I drank tea and other hot drinks all day long, and was still cold. Within three days of my first remedy, I warmed up. I craved ice cold drinks like mad and since then, have rarely wanted hot ones. I stopped covering up with the quilt, and began throwing off my sweater, even in air-conditioned places where I used to be ever so cold.

There used to be several homeopathic hospitals and schools in America in the 1800s, and life insurance was cheaper for home-opathy patients because they were healthier and lived longer than those who used conventional medical treatments. But the medical authorities, feeling threatened, made sure doctors' licenses were removed if they or their families saw homeopaths.

Samuel Hahnemann is a great historical figure and in Washington DC, USA, there is a statue of him in recognition of his contribution to healing around the world. More than 200 years after his first proving, there are many colleges and centres in different countries where students can learn this powerful, yet gentle, alternative medicine.

And to think there are still people in the world who doubt its validity. Their excuse for this is that there is no scientific explanation for how it works, but of course, there is.

However, there is no science to explain one of the most bizarre experiences of my life. It would become an experience that unlocked the door to something so mysterious, yet so powerful, to this day I struggle to understand it.

Chapter Twenty-Five

One day, in 1995, I was sitting and talking with a friend. During the conversation, he mentioned that one of his knees was extremely painful. Under normal circumstances, I'd have simply offered a compassionate word or two, especially because of my own painful knees, and no doubt we would have moved on to discuss something else.

But on that occasion, somewhere deep down inside me, I heard quiet words, giving me instructions. Put my hand here, imagine this, put my hand there, do that...it was all a bit odd, to say the least, but I continued to take direction and did as I was told. In the middle of it, my friend asked, "What are you doing?"

"I don't know," I replied. "I have no idea. Hang on a minute."

Patiently, he let me carry on. I could feel a sort of toxic sludge energy being pulled into my hand and once that subsided, I was given different instructions that were about putting healing energy into his knee. A few minutes later, I "knew" that I was finished and put my hands back in my lap. I looked at my friend, who was staring at me with his mouth open. "What did you do?" he asked, looking bewildered.

"I don't know, really. I think that was supposed to help but it's never happened before."

"The pain is gone."

I was shocked. "Gone? Not just better? Actually gone?"

"Yeah, gone. It doesn't hurt any more. It was terrible before you started, and it's terrible most of the time. And now it's fine. How did you know what to do?" he asked, obviously as incredulous as I was.

I had no answer for him. And I knew I was meant to do more of this. I'd got out of bed that day, expecting it to be just like every other day, tending to my children and my life. By the time I went to bed again that night, I had been shown how to use the powerful creative energy that exists throughout the universe, and to direct it to flow through my body, out the palms of my hands (interestingly, as per Tai Chi wisdom, which I did not know until many years later), and into my friend for the purposes of healing.

To tell you how this ultimately changed my life would require a whole other book, so I must stick to the topic at hand. Clearly, there had been a reason why I was shown how to use this powerful energy. I began to practice on my friends when they complained of various aches and pains — although I hasten to add, it was always with their permission because to heal without it is taking away their free will. Very quickly, I discovered that I could detect exactly where people were having problems, firstly by tuning in psychically, and then by holding my hand about an inch or two away from their bodies.

For example, if someone said he had back pain, without actually touching him I would scan the energy field over his entire back with my hand, locating the areas that felt different in a way that I cannot describe. Placing my hand on those areas, I would ask "Is it here?" Always the answer was "Yes." Then I would do what I lovingly referred to as "my zappy thing" and the pain would disappear.

I began to experiment with this ability and it wasn't long before I discovered that it worked not only for physical complaints, but emotional troubles, too, such as anxiety and depression. At some point, I decided to see if I could do it at a distance, tuning in and focusing on a person and essentially doing the same general steps but visualising them in my mind. I couldn't have been more shocked when I discovered that **that** worked, too. I was still struggling to believe I could really do this at all, never mind when I wasn't anywhere near the person who was getting the healing. No one was more surprised than I was on every single one of those occasions because whatever the ailment, there was always dramatic improvement or complete healing.

The only exceptions to the rule were these: sometimes it worked on my children, and sometimes it did not. And it never worked when I did it on myself. It would take many years before I figured out the reasons for these inconsistencies.

In 2005, a woman who acted as my agent, and who organised a book-signing for me, went out on a limb without consulting me. Ringing me to tell me about the book-signing, she said, "And I've arranged a healing event for you the following night at the same place."

I was horrified. I had been doing this healing for ten years at that point but had never done it "on demand." I had only ever done it here and there, as and when the mood felt right, and in the presence of family or friends when it wouldn't have mattered if it hadn't been successful. I had only done it if I thought I had the energy and focus for it. I had no idea what would happen in a public venue. I didn't want to disappoint anyone, nor did I want to look like a complete and utter fool.

I didn't want to cancel; it would have been unprofessional. I bit the bullet and decided to just go for it and hope for the best. I consoled myself with the knowledge that it was taking place in a small village, and figured only two or three people would turn up, if any.

Famous last words...the place was packed. All seats were taken, whilst many people stood leaning against walls or in doorways, wherever they could. Some of them were hecklers but I was not deterred. And how wonderful it was when I gave them their turn, and with no hints from them, I told them or showed them where there was pain or discomfort in their bodies, and then made it vanish.

One man in particular had been quite loud about giving me grief in the hours before it was his turn. "Yeah, sure, I'll just *bet* you can fix what's wrong with me!" he sneered, over and over again. I was delighted to see the stunned look on his face when I detected the problems and removed the pain with which he'd been suffering every day for years. In front of everyone, he was only too happy to take back his unkind comments and say he had been completely wrong about me. I saw him from time to time in the village over the next five or six years, and always stopped to have a word. His pain never did return.

On that healing night, October 26, 2005, I saw approximately 30 people back-to-back from 7.30 p.m. till 1.30 a.m. Looking back, I don't know how I was able to do that. Until that night, I had always felt quite drained after several minutes of healing, never mind six hours without a break. I must admit that as soon as the last person left, suddenly I felt as though I had been filled with ice water, and at the same time, I was absolutely overwhelmed with exhaustion.

That night, I was shocked and delighted to learn a very important lesson. My abilities as a healer were far more powerful than I could have imagined. Still, as I drifted off to sleep, I choked back tears, wondering why I could not heal myself.

I had been a die-hard homeopath for many years, having witnessed its miraculous healing power both personally and professionally. And there was the 1995 discovery of my natural ability to heal, and various other related forms of "energy healing" that I have experienced since then. Just when I thought I had seen everything, I stumbled upon something even more powerful. It is so powerful, in fact, that an inoperable 3-inch cancerous tumour on a woman's bladder disappeared in a matter of minutes.

Available to view online, this incredible video, created by Master Luke Chan, was filmed in a "medicine-less" hospital in China. People from all over the world go to ZhongShan, China, to attend Master Chan's 25-day courses in Qigong, a practice that dates back approximately 7,000 years. Practitioners and "students" (not "patients") create the feeling as if the healing is complete and in the past. There are other steps prior to this, of course, ensuring that the "student" is also eating, exercising and breathing in ways that maximise the healing and empowering flow of Qi energy. In this video of the woman with bladder cancer, she is surrounded by three practitioners, who are chanting in unison. Loosely translated, they are essentially saying that she has already been fully healed.

The secret lies in much more than mere words. It is in the emotion and belief behind them. The practitioners and the woman are all feeling the feeling that she is completely healed. They are not thinking about making her cancer go away. They feel deeply that it is already so and as we watch the live action on an ultrasound monitor, we see the tumour vanish in less than three minutes. It begins with the belief, which is fueled by the emotion that goes with it. It sounds incredible, but as we have seen in the information about Dissociative Identity Disorder, it is quite possible for the mind to create or disintegrate tumours at will, and without the help of anyone else. All it takes is an absolute, right-through-to-the-core belief.

As I said near the beginning of this book, my search for healing led me down a very long and twisted road, ultimately ending right back at my own feet with the discovery that I could heal myself.

And perhaps something in this book can help you heal yourself, too.

But where do you start? You've waded through a wealth of tools and information within these pages. How do you put it all together?

With one more piece of the puzzle.

Chapter Twenty-Six

The piece that ties all of this together is actually very simple. It's meditation. Don't let that word put you off if it's a sticking point for you. Some people say, "I've tried meditating a million times and I just can't do it!" Don't panic. To "meditate" simply means to contemplate, reflect, or ponder. What I'm talking about is straightforward: spending time on your own, uninterrupted, without any disturbances, eyes closed, and focusing on particular affirmations, images, or thoughts. There are almost as many ways to meditate as there are people in the world, so just do it your way—it will work fine.

You may recall in Chapter 5, I discussed the health benefits of meditation, and that people who meditate regularly tend to live longer and have fewer health problems than those who do not. Using everything you've learned in this book in your meditations will be some of the most powerful, concentrated work you can do. But what you think about outside of meditation time is just as important because your subconscious is always, always listening. I like to think of those "in-between thoughts" as mini-meditations. For instance, if you take a few moments here and there throughout the day to reinforce healing thoughts, or if you're at the sink doing the washing up and notice your mind drifting to your health, take the opportunity to replace any negative thoughts with positive ones. That's a mini-meditation.

One of my favourite ways to meditate is during my morning walk (weather permitting, of course). My mantra changes depending on my mood, but throughout the walk I repeat various statements to myself. It might go something like this: "I weigh less than ten stone. I look and feel like I'm in my 20s. Every single cell in my body has regenerated and become perfectly healed and strong. I am a power-house of youthful energy and strength. I am in perfect health and balance on all levels of my being."

Sometimes my statements focus on specific areas of my body, like my heart being perfectly pink and strong, or my kidneys being ener-gised and functioning in perfect balance. I get so absorbed in visual-izing my fully healed body that I often don't notice I've walked a few miles.

Repeating thoughts like these always makes me feel empowered and strong. There's so much positive energy in these words; it fills every part of me and sets me up for a wonderful day.

I've never been a fan of books that give a blow-by-blow guide to meditation, walking you through each step, one image or instruction at a time. If you're meant to have your eyes closed and be relaxing, how can you follow along with the book at the same time? How can you truly relax and focus on meditating if you're trying to remember several paragraphs of detailed instructions?

I don't know your exact needs, ailments, or issues, so I can only provide an outline—you must do the "colouring-in." I've given you plenty of ideas and tools to create your own healing meditations. You can make the process as simple or as detailed as you like.

The most important thing is to **use only positive language** in your meditations. Your subconscious does not accept negatives. Words like "not," "never," or "don't" won't be heard as intended. For example, if you say, "I am not sick," your subconscious hears, "I am sick."

Choose your words carefully and phrase everything positively: "I am in perfect health." Think about the consequences of each word, because your subconscious will take them literally. Don't focus on illness—focus on perfect health, strength, and vitality.

You can imagine little soldiers running through your body or bloodstream, making sure you are well. You might picture a fire-breathing dragon torching tumours until they disintegrate, or even imagine Steven Seagal taking out the "bad guy."

You can imagine angels filling you with healing light or energy, fairies sprinkling you with healing fairy dust, or any number of other images that work for you. As long as you remain positive in your language and focused on the outcome you hope for, it doesn't really matter which route you take with your meditations. All of them start at the same point — your thoughts — and are moving toward the same destination: your healing. The more time and energy you spend in a focused meditation, the more it may help.

Remember that whether you are meditating or not, every thought you allow or choose is creating neurotransmitters that send chemical messages to every cell in your body, and they will respond accordingly. Don't panic if unexpected negative thoughts drift through your mind. Simply let them go and replace them with positive, empowering ones. Don't be hard on yourself for having a negative thought; that only creates more negative energy and can make things feel worse. Just let the thought pass and gently refocus on something positive.

I see this all the time when I teach meditation classes. In the early days, students often become upset with themselves when their minds drift from the focus. It's the same when I've worked with counselling clients who try to eliminate all negative thoughts. Old habits of self-criticism flare up, and they chastise themselves for it. But in doing so —whether in meditation or regular thinking — they often end up spinning further off track, which only adds to frustration.

We cannot control random thoughts that enter our minds uninvited. But what we do with them is entirely up to us. If you choose to dwell on them, you give them strength, creating corresponding chemical signals in the body — positive or negative. Over time, however, as you continue regular work to shift your belief systems, you may notice that unbidden negative thoughts gradually decrease. Thoughts are a natural byproduct of our beliefs, and beliefs are shaped by our thoughts. As mentioned earlier, the subconscious is always listening, always active, and always sending up signals based on what it has been fed. So if you find yourself receiving negative or self-destructive messages, you can try feeding it more positive thoughts instead.

You've been given a lot of information in this book. Now it's time to start incorporating it into your life, and you may want to consider what it is you hope to achieve. Try to create a vision for yourself — your health, your energy, the things you'd like to be able to do. Once you can imagine it clearly in your mind, you have a starting point.

Perhaps you can remember a time when you were in good health, felt energetic, and were mostly free of physical complaints, anxiety, or depression. If you can, hold onto those memories. Reconnect with how it felt to have that kind of freedom. Recall how easily you could move about, do what you wanted, and feel happy and at peace with your life, despite its usual little glitches.

Perhaps you have never felt well, or it's been so long that you can't remember how it felt. You are not alone; many people are in the same position. In that case, try to create a clear picture in your mind of what you would like to accomplish and how you would like to feel.

Either way, it's like setting out on a journey — you can't plan your route unless you know your destination.

I hope, as I suggested in Chapter 3, that you've been making notes while reading this book, keeping track of key points and making a checklist of what you want to change. Perhaps you've even started incorporating some of my suggestions and noticed some small improvements.

Either way, write down what you plan to achieve. Be specific;

merely thinking about your goal isn't enough. Create an image in your mind that represents what you want to accomplish, and write it down. Using the written word helps solidify the image and desire — and may give your efforts a little extra power.

You may find, too, in the coming days and weeks that you think of things you would like to add to the list of changes you want to make, which can only give you more reason to focus on your goal. Look at your list every day. Keep it where you can see it easily and often. Focus on that picture in your mind that represents a healthy, happy and fulfilled "you." This will help to keep your eye on where you want to be. When doubts creep in, just conjure up that image, focus on it, and insist that success is your only option.

Having sorted out your destination, now you must plan the route you will take to get there. Please bear in mind that I am not a doctor and of course, even if I were, I do not know your particular circumstances. I can only share my personal experiences and what I have learned. I can tell you what has worked for me, and what I have found to be true, based on my investigations. You must take responsibility for your own health and depending on your circumstances, you may wish to consult your doctor or other qualified medical professional before embarking on this journey, and discuss any concerns that might arise on either side.

Be prepared to make changes gradually; you cannot be expected to give yourself a complete overhaul in every way all at once or you will set yourself up for failure. As long as you are keeping yourself focused on where you want to be, and you are taking steps toward that goal every day, you will continue to make progress. Don't beat yourself up for being human and not being able to go from A to Z immediately. It took time for you to become as ill as you are. It will take time for you to create new habits and to become well. This cannot happen overnight. It is a process and should be seen as such.

Start with the basics. If you plant seeds in cold, dry rocks in the dead of winter when they require nutrient-rich soil in the warmth of spring, they will never take root and grow. If you do not provide the best possible conditions for your physical health and wellbeing, you will never quite get there. So you must begin by taking stock of everything to do with the physical aspects of your life. Be honest; no one has to see the list but you. The more honest you are, the more you will be able to see what needs changing. The only one who benefits — or doesn't — from your choices is you.

Write down what you usually eat and drink. It may help for you to keep track of everything that goes into your mouth for a while, at least a week or two, as you may surprise yourself and discover that your diet is far worse than you realised. I would strongly urge you to at least read about the blood type diet and discover why certain foods and drinks are particularly harmful or beneficial to you, as this might help you to understand why it is worth giving this diet a try for a while. But even if you choose not to do that, it is imperative that you eat as many fresh, whole foods as possible — preferably organic — and to eliminate or reduce your consumption of processed and junk foods.

I am not suggesting that you be militant and cut out everything "naughty". There is nothing wrong with having a little treat now and then. But bear in mind that what you put into your body is what you will get out of it. The higher the quality of food and beverages you consume, the more your body will appreciate it and respond positively. Yes, it takes more than a healthful, balanced diet to be well, but you must begin there. You cannot put loads of fat, sugar, and refined, processed foods into your body, complete with all sorts of toxic chemical ingredients you cannot pronounce, and expect that you will recover or be healthy and strong.

Look at what you are drinking every day, and how much. Be sure to have several glasses of water and use decaffeinated beverages wherever possible. Caffeine dehydrates the body, jangles the nerves and in general, is perceived by the body as a poison (which is why people can die from caffeine overdose).

If you are a coffee-drinker, try to limit yourself to a cup or two a day, or try replacing it with another hot drink such as the delicious mineral whey I mentioned, or perhaps something like Postum. Tea should also be decaffeinated, and if you cannot buy a decaf version of your favourite tea, you can remove the caffeine yourself. Pour the hot water over your tea bags or leaves, and let it stand for about 30 seconds (much longer than that and you will lose a lot of the flavour so be careful). Drain and proceed as usual to make your tea. Most of the caffeine comes out of the leaves within those first several seconds, as do the bitter tannins so you end up with a more delicious cup of tea that does not affect you adversely.

Many people enjoy the odd alcoholic beverage — or a few — with no noticeable consequences. Some authorities say a little of it is actually good for us. Don't worry, I am not going to suggest you never touch it again if it's something you like. I used to have a couple of glasses of wine every evening, simply because I loved the taste. It seemed a terrible thing to have to give up this simple pleasure when I moved to Canada and could not afford it. Interestingly, I discovered that the longer I went without it, the less I wanted it, which may have been a happy - and unexpected — "side effect" of my self-healing project.

Now, I find that at times when I could have wine, I would rather have water. It's not even a conscious choice. It's as though now that my body has been exposed to such a positive environment, healthful foods and so on, it wants more of the same. It knows instinctively that alcohol is a poison in the same way I have become averse to cigarettes.

At any rate, you must decide for yourself what you'd to do about having alcohol. This entire self-healing exercise is about looking at habits and finding ways in which you can give your body its best chance physically to respond to the other healing steps you will be taking. Alcohol is quite toxic to the body in anything more than very small amounts. There is a reason why people who drink too much alcohol become "in-**_toxic_**-ated", and sometimes even die of alcohol poisoning, or end up with cirrhosis of the liver, dementia, and a host of other nasty (and entirely unnecessary) problems.

Smoking —well, we don't really need to discuss that one now, do we? You will never be particularly well if you smoke. No matter how perfect your diet or how much you exercise, or how balanced your life is in other ways, you will be loading yourself up with toxins and poisons so that eventually, your body will be overwhelmed by them. If you are a regular smoker, you probably hack and cough a lot, as your lungs struggle to eliminate the black sticky mess that is accumulating in them and making it hard for them to get oxygen into your bloodstream. I don't need to tell you about the damage you're doing; you've heard it all before.

I know how tough it can be to stop; been there, done that off and on for a while myself, as you know. Thankfully, with all of the other healing work I have done, finally the desire to smoke has completely left me. As I did not smoke for most of my life, I am still surprised that I took it up at mid-life, and had an on-again, off-again, love/hate relationship with it for a few years. Sometimes I think it was a subconscious death wish because I had become so fed up with my ill health and all the rest of my life struggles; there can only ever be self-destruction at the heart of the desire to smoke. I am so grateful that as a result of my self-healing work, I know I will never smoke again.

If you smoke and are having trouble stopping, you might like to make it easier on yourself and try my "**Stop Smoking NOW With Hypnosis**" audio, which is available for purchase on my website. It's not just for cigarette-smokers; it can work if you are smoking pipes or cigars — or anything other than tobacco (wink, wink), for that matter.

You can put all kinds of good stuff into your body but if you're putting poison into it, too, that's going to massively impact your ability to reach your goal for good health. You know this already. But are you ready to do something about it?

Chapter Twenty-Seven

Another important consideration in healing yourself is to research supplements, particularly high potency antioxidants and certain vitamins as recommended in Dr Ray Strand's book or by other qualified professionals. Or you may wish to check out ProArgi-9+, which may significantly improve, or even eliminate whatever is ailing you. It has certainly made an incredibly powerful and noticeable difference in my own health, my overall strength, and energy levels —and there is another benefit that I had not anticipated.

As you may recall from the information I shared with you about this product, it has been discovered that the real cause of cardiovascular disease is inflammation of the blood vessels. Interestingly, the relationship between heart disease and periodontal disease has become more clearer than ever. Professionals are now saying that if you have one, your risk of the other increases greatly.

According to Dr David Cochran, DDS, PhD, President of the American Academy of Periodontology and Chair of the Department of Periodontics at the University of Texas Health Science Center, "Both periodontal disease and cardiovascular disease are inflammatory diseases, and inflammation is the common mechanism that connects them."

There is speculation about why this relationship exists but in my opinion, it seems quite obvious. When you look at gums, they are almost like looking under your skin. The blood vessels are right there, close to the surface. It seems to me that when we have inflamed, swollen, bleeding gums, we're just seeing a sample of what is going on in the rest of the vascular system. The only difference between the blood vessels in your gums and the others that are elsewhere in your body is that you get a more "up close and personal" look at the ones in your mouth.

So don't ignore this very important aspect of your health. It can be too easy to think about teeth as being separate from the rest of you, but they are just as much a part of you as your bones and the rest of your mouth are. Again, you must use a holistic approach in self-healing; all parts of you are connected to one another. Be sure to sort out any overdue dental issues and take care of your teeth and gums diligently, as they are just as important as every other part of your body in terms of your overall health.

It is especially important to get yourself to the dentist if you have been experiencing an unusual amount of stress. A while after my move back to Canada, I had to sort out finding a dentist. When I went for my first appointment, the woman who was going to clean my teeth asked all of those usual "new patient" questions, like when I had last seen a dentist. This brought up the subject of England, and I became weepy. Feeling ever so foolish, I told her that the move had been the most painful and traumatic experience of my life and that I was still struggling to adjust. I explained that it had been a terribly stressful time, to say the least, and that I really hated being in Calgary - and away from the only place I had ever felt was "home".

When she finished poking around in my mouth, I was horrified to learn that I had a borderline case of periodontal disease in the area where I have six crowns — and this, despite taking reasonably good care of my teeth and gums. I told her that my gums had never been the same since getting the crowns, which she advised was because there's metal under the outer part of a crown, and it irritates the gums. Had I known this, I never would have got the crowns. But 30-odd years ago, my dentist hadn't said a word about potential troubles.

She also told me that stress can overwhelm the immune system — no surprise, but definitely not helpful with an already-compromised area. However, what I did not know was that if the stress gets bad enough, the immune system can become so weak, it can no longer fight the bacteria that attack the gums. To be honest, this was quite frightening. I had to wonder: if my immune system could not even manage that, how on earth was it keeping me free of cancer, worsening heart disease and heaven knows what else?

Thankfully, at least the problem with my gums was still reversible — *just* — but it had never been that bad in the past, even though I had endured ongoing high levels of stress as far back as I could remember. Apparently, leaving England — and all that had happened since — had taken an even greater toll on my physical health than I realised.

In your pursuit of healing, reaching and maintaining a healthy weight is also something to consider. If you believe that you should either gain or lose some weight, find an online BMI (body mass index) calculator that will figure out the healthy weight range for your age, height and gender in a matter of seconds, Or speak to a doctor. If a change is required, approach it sensibly and gradually.

It is not good to be too thin, and of course being overweight carries risks as well. There are all sorts of weight loss programs to try but remember, slow and steady is always going to be better than anything drastic. Rapid weight loss is quite dangerous and is usually self-defeating, as your body thinks it is in starvation mode and produces fat-storing enzymes in an effort to protect you.

The only way to successfully take off pounds and keep them off is to change your lifestyle. It is about learning a new way of looking at food and paying attention to what - and how much — you are putting into your mouth. Eat less and do more. Crank up your metabolism early in the day with some exercise, and keep it cranked by eating something at least every three hours.

By the way, skipping meals is a great way to *keep* all the weight you wish you could drop. Your body thinks you're starving and produces extra fat-storing enzymes, just to keep you safe. Virtually everything you put in your mouth will be stored as fat.

And while we're on the subject of weight reducing tactics, an easy one is to drink oolong tea with meals, or just after, as it prevents the absorption of fat and the formation of triglycerides. When fats and sugars hit the liver and small intestine, they are turned into triglycerides, which we need as a source of energy to keep us alive.

However, when there are too many, they make their way into the bloodstream and are deposited into fat cells. Oolong tea activates the enzyme in the body that is responsible for dissolving triglycerides, thereby reducing the body's ability to store excess fat.

It's also another warrior in the battle against free radicals and slowing the age process, it helps prevent liver spots and wrinkles, and its polyphenols even help reduce or prevent tooth decay. Personally, not being a big tea-drinker, I'm not keen on the taste of oolong by itself, but it is quite refreshing with a bit of fresh lemon juice squeezed into it. I make sure I have it at least a couple of times a day, particularly if I've eaten a fatty meal.

On the subject of weight loss, because of my history with anorexia, I feel compelled to bring up the subject of eating disorders, which ironically have absolutely nothing to do with weight or with food. They have everything to do with anxiety and huge stress around not feeling "good enough." Excessive anxiety in childhood is just one of the many causes of eating disorders, which always have their roots in issues of self-esteem, self-love, self-worth and especially, issues of control.

There are countless books available to purchase online (where you can read reviews) or in bookshops. The one that began to unravel my anorexia nightmare and helped me to understand why I was starving myself was a brilliant little book called "The Golden Cage, the Enigma of Anorexic Nervosa" by Hilde Bruch, MD.

It was around the time that I was addressing my addiction, anxiety disorder, panic attacks and obsessive-compulsive disorder (OCD) — all of which are just different spokes on the same wheel — and anorexia is another. As it is a kind of anxiety disorder, between that little book and what I was learning about how my thoughts affected anxiety, I began to see results immediately. Over the following months, there was ongoing improvement until eventually my nine-year battle with starving myself had ended. And I won.

If you are struggling with an eating disorder, or in fact, feel overwhelmed by emotional wounds that are causing you pain in any way, you may also wish to consider seeing a reputable psychologist, as they can help you dig out the roots of the problems and get you on a path of healing them. Even just a few sessions could give you a big boost toward getting you started down that road.

What about drugs? Are you at the chemist's too often, taking prescription meds that you would rather not take, or are no longer sure you even need? Are you always buying over-the-counter aids for sleep, stomach upset, headaches or other ailments? Obviously, prescription medications need to be discussed with whoever prescribed them for you, but perhaps it is worth doing. Sometimes people are not even sure what they are taking or why, and occasionally they discover that they can come off medications, or the dosage can be lowered.

Once you have closely examined all foods, drinks and other substances that you are putting into your body, take a look at how much exercise you are getting and write it in your notebook. I understand that you may be severely restricted, perhaps even bed-ridden or wheelchair-bound. But whatever your situation, be honest with yourself about what you are doing in terms of any sort of activity, especially if you know you are already able to do much more than you are doing. Again, no one has to see this list but you.

When you have seen where you are, then you can see where

you're going. Set your intention for the changes you want to make, even if they seem impossible to you now. We will get to the rest of the 'how to' shortly. For now, let's just stick with what you are doing presently, and what you would like to be able to do in the future. Remember, I was terribly restricted by my heart problem, as well as pain and dislocations in my knee and hip for years, until I began incorporating all of these "puzzle pieces" into my life. It was not long before I was zooming along at a very brisk pace with no trouble at all.

It is essential to be active in whatever ways you can manage. If all you can do is make circles with your hands or arms, or move your torso or your feet, then do it as often as possible. If you can only get out for a 5-10 minute walk or leisurely stroll, do it. Turn on some music and dance around your home. Do several trips up and down your stairs, if you have them, or if someone rings you for a long chat, make good use of the time by walking as briskly as possible around a large room or up and down a long hallway whilst talking on the phone (another favourite of mine if the weather is miserable).

If those don't work for you, there are countless DVDs, YouTube videos, apps etc. available that will teach you how to do yoga, Tai Chi, dance workouts and all sorts of other physical activities. Many of them are geared toward people who have physical limitations and there are loads of them out there for beginners.

If you can move parts of your body — even if it hurts, but will not do any actual harm — then you must move them — every day. I am reminded of "The Miracle Man", Morris Goodman. If you have seen Rhonda Byrne's documentary film, "The Secret", you will know his story.

In March of 1981, when he was 35 years old, he was in a plane crash, breaking his neck in two places and leaving him with a crushed spinal cord. Every single muscle in his body was completely destroyed, as was his diaphragm, making it impossible for him to breathe on his own. He could not speak; his larynx was crushed. He could not swallow. His liver, kidneys, bladder and bowel did not function. All he could move were his eyelids. He was able to blink;

that's it. He was not expected to survive, and if by some miracle he did that, he would most certainly never walk again.

Goodman would not accept this. Awake and aware of his surroundings and his situation, but unable to move or communicate, apart from blinking, the days were mighty long. He busied himself with recovering, willing himself to be well. He swore that he would walk out of that hospital on his own steam by Christmas. And miracle of miracles, he did it. Against all odds, he had survived, learned how to breathe using abdominal muscles, as his diaphragm was (and still is) non-functional. Eventually, he was able to eat, and to say a few words. He walked out of hospital, unassisted, on November 13, 1981.

That was only a beginning point. His recovery was long, slow and painful. But he did it.

If that doesn't inspire you to work toward getting yourself up and moving, nothing will.

Chapter Twenty-Eight

Once you have taken stock of any diet, exercise and other lifestyle changes that need to be made on a physical level, it is time to move on to making changes on an energetic level. First, consider your environment. Perhaps after reading about EMFs, you have already made some changes in that regard. If not, this is as good a time as any to go back to Chapter 21 and review the information and suggestions about how you can minimise your exposure to electromagnetic waves.

Look around your home. Does it need a clear-out? A de-clutter? Every single item in your home is holding energy, and not all of it is good. You may find it helpful to do some reading about feng shui and see what you think about it. There are various ways to practice feng shui, so investigate all the options before making a decision.

Because of the serene and tranquil energy in my home, many people have become interested in feng shui. They have found that even making some small changes, or just doing feng shui treatments in one or two rooms has made a noticeable difference to the overall feeling in their homes.

Whether or not you decide to give feng shui a try, it is always a good idea to go through every nook and cranny in your home with some regularity and get rid of anything you don't need or want. Personally, that's one of my favourite things to do. It always feels so good; for me, it's like a thorough cleansing of the soul. I have found that by tackling small areas on a regular basis, it does not become an overwhelming "spring-cleaning" task.

Your inner world is reflected in your environment. If your home is cluttered and chaotic, you can bet that you feel this way on the inside. As you are on a journey of self-healing, it involves self-evaluation, clearing out the old, making way for the new. Doing this in your physical environment is an excellent way to help you in this process.

Consider everything in your environment, everything you "take in" that is around you. Look at it with a view to uncovering all the places in which there is negativity lurking. What do you watch on the telly? What do you read? What kinds of conversations do you usually have? Wherever possible, cut out anything that is regarded as negative input. Suspenseful, anxiety-producing films, disturbing television shows, newspapers loaded with terrible stories around the world, persistently negative people who spend more time complaining and grumbling than anything...

There are numerous ways in which you can expose yourself to the harmful effects of negative energy. The more you think about it, watch it, listen to it and participate in it, the more damage it is doing to you on all levels of your being. It may be subtle and not overtly noticeable, but its effects can be profound and long lasting.

What about the people with whom you associate? This one can be tricky, of course, depending on the nature of the relationships that are negative, but it is worth finding ways to make changes wherever you are able. Perhaps some relationships need to end or you need to set clear boundaries about the amount of time spent with those people, or about the content of the conversations. Do what you must; your health is at stake and if there are people around you who are thwarting your efforts to be well, then you have a right, and in fact an obligation to yourself, to avoid, reduce or eliminate their influence as much as you can.

In some cases, you may need to become quite militant about what you will and won't tolerate. When others aren't respectful of you, your needs or your health, you may just have to put your foot down — at least until you are well. If they don't respect you, do you *really* need to worry a whole lot about whether they'll be upset about your decision? Are they the ones who will have to live in your skin and put up with the repercussions for your health?

Nope. You have a right to surround yourself with respect and kindness — *especially* while you work on healing yourself.

There's so much more that I could say on this and many related subjects but they are well beyond the scope of this book. For now, let's stick to the more specific ways in which you can contribute to healing yourself.

Aside from the lifestyle, physical and environmental factors that affect your health, the rest of your self-healing journey will begin in your mind, as your ability to heal yourself is directly related to the thoughts you choose and the beliefs that they nurture or create. This is where meditation comes in. If you're like most people, many of your thoughts and beliefs have contributed to making making you ill and therefore, changing them while meditating can help to make you well.

And when you do "go there" with negative thoughts about yourself, don't beat yourself up about it; you're human. We've all got the ability to think negatively about ourselves or put ourselves down in moments of frustration. It's in our DNA. Throw in all those supposedly "perfect" people living great lives on social media and it's easy to have your self-esteem take a hit. A lot of it happens without us even noticing. So whatever we can do to counteract those beliefs and deliberately deposit a bunch of good stuff into the subconscious is going to help.

This can be a powerful first step in your healing and for some reason, it's a step that in my experience, people will say is difficult or impossible before they've even tried it. That's only because they have not learned how to train their minds. It requires a bit of discipline to think the thoughts you want, and to keep drop-kicking the other ones to the curb, but it can be done. The good news is that the more you do it, the easier it gets. You might want to check out mindfulness meditations online, as this is one of the most useful tools in training your mind.

Certainly, you could see a reputable and well-qualified hypnotist for just such a short-cut. It would give you a head start in changing the beliefs that are locked away in your subconscious and not doing you any favours. You can also do it yourself. Depending on what needs changing and how you approach it, you could notice results fairly quickly.

For example, if you're having a miserable day and feeling like everything is going wrong, stop yourself for a moment. Quit thinking about all the things that suck and start thinking about some of the good stuff in your life, or the things that are going well. Count a blessing or two or three. Imagine looking inside a kaleidoscope. Now imagine turning it ever so slightly. You get a whole new picture, right? All of the same little bits are still in there, but it looks completely different. Your perspective works the same way.

Life is like that, too. Every bad day, bad moment, bad experience, all of it can be viewed as though you are looking into a kaleidoscope. As miserable as things might be in your life, there is always something good somewhere. Change your perspective when you are having negative thoughts and see how quickly your mood shifts. It's a great experiment to prove that changing your thoughts will change how you feel.

Hopefully, you've already been making an effort to shove aside any negative thoughts and replace them with positive ones. Whatever the topic, whatever you are doing, and with the company you're keeping, you must do your best to keep your thoughts as positive as possible. As you are working on healing yourself, it will be most helpful for you to consider everything you think and do in terms of the energy involved. Is it a drain on your energy? Is it bringing positive energy into your days? Do you feel exhausted or uplifted after being with certain people or doing certain activities?

That's one of the quickest ways to figure out what needs to stay and what needs to go. Obviously, sometimes there are obligations or situations we can't change and they aren't exactly bringing us joy. This is even more reason to deliberately insert positive thoughts, people, and experiences into our lives wherever possible.

You might recall what I wrote in Chapter 12 about the long-term damage we suffer during periods of chronic stress. While we're in "fight or flight", the growth response is inhibited, leaving us unable to produce energy, yet we're using loads of it to cope with our perceived stressors. To say we "burn out" is more appropriate than we probably realise. This physiological situation is further confirmation that we're not designed to tolerate anything negative.

I am about to make another one of those statements that might make you want to throw rocks at my house. I'm going to say it anyway because it's the truth, and it can help you enormously, if you give it a chance to settle inside your soul.

We will only have stress if we *believe in* stress.

Please contemplate that for a moment before you continue...

And before I go on, I understand that sometimes we have to deal with tragic and extremely difficult situations. Let's leave those aside and focus on the more usual, day-to-day kinds of issues that we say are stressful. Busy life, lots to do, jam-packed schedule, kids driving you nuts, partner, too, a jerk for a boss, idiots in traffic...

Yep, they can all feel stressful. And it can help you feel better if you work toward changing how you view them.

In dealing with those challenging parts of your life, the language you choose will make all the difference in the world. This is one of the first places you can make a change in your health, and as I have said already, it begins by changing your thoughts about them. If you believe these issues are stressful, this produces stressful thoughts, cranks up your cortisol and adrenaline, wreaking havoc on your body and loading your mind and emotions with negativity.

The more you stay in those thoughts, the more you validate the beliefs and perpetuate the problem. That chicken-and-egg thing again.

Taking one of those stressful moments at a time, you can let go of the thoughts that aren't helpful. You can choose ones that are more calming or supportive. You can have a positive outlook and instead of seeing how awful something is right now, tell yourself you're getting through it and working on solutions.

The more you choose calming, forward-thinking, positive thoughts in those bumpy moments, the better you'll feel. It might not change the jerk boss or the grumpy partner or your financial problems, but it'll definitely help you cope with them. It can help you see everything in a more balanced way or find solutions or see the bright spots if you're not immersing yourself in how stressful and upsetting it is.

I've survived a lot of trauma and crises; I am no stranger to "stress." I only wish that through most of it, I'd known this little nugget of truth because I can tell you, since I stumbled upon it, it's changed the way I view difficult situations that the universe throws at me. I get through them so much better than I did when I viewed them as "stressful."

I'm not saying I never get upset or feel stressed, but I'm much more aware of those moments and it's now second nature to shift from those thoughts into the ones that serve my health and wellbeing. I don't stay on the hamster wheel of fearful, angry, or worrying thoughts. I skip over to a positive lane and into thoughts that allow me a sense of control over myself, my life, and whatever the issue is that has put itself in my path. It is easier to stay calm and focused now, and this makes all the difference in the world when I need to keep my wits about me and deal with a problem.

Telling yourself you are "so stressed!" does nothing to make you feel better. In fact, it only makes you feel worse. Such thoughts will send all those damaging "stress hormones" throughout your body, jacking up your blood pressure, heart rate, anxiety level etc. Negativity never going to do you any favours; it's only ever harmful. The biggest problem we have is that we are so used to its presence in many areas of our lives, we don't even see it anymore. It has become an insidious, toxic killer.

A wonderful place to begin incorporating positive energy into your life is with a piece of paper taped to a glass jug of water, courtesy of Dr Emoto's work. Think about the qualities you want in your life, such as joy, peace, gratitude, or you could address your emotional wounds as I did, and write whatever it is you need to heal them, eg. self-love, forgiveness, etc. Or perhaps simply write "healing" or "perfect health". Use permanent marker or indelible ink to prevent smudging if you get the paper wet when refilling the jug. If nothing else, the very act of doing this and focusing on these qualities while you are drinking the water is still bound to have a positive effect on how you feel.

During the early stages of this project, I went a step further and considered my body to *be* the vessel that contains water — because it does. I sat comfortably for quite some time, eyes closed, and focused on the energy of these words permeating the water in every cell of my body:

"I have let go of the pain of my past, and the hurt caused by others. No one has the power to hurt me; I can choose how I respond to the actions of others. I choose to see only good in every experience I have ever had, or will ever have. It's all for my benefit.

"I forgive everyone who has ever caused pain in my life (I focused on a few in particular that I was still allowing to affect me). I forgive them because they are not perfect and did the best they could in their circumstances, and because I would want them to forgive me, too.

"I forgive myself for my weaknesses, my mistakes, and the poor choices I've made. I choose to learn from them and let them go. I forgive myself for the hurt I've caused others. I let go of my guilt. I did the best I could in those circumstances with the tools I had at the time, and I'm doing my best to choose better every day."

"I let go of any subconscious need for my illness. I let go of the need for my symptoms (I listed several). I let go of the need for restriction."

I found myself feeling lighter and happier after focusing on these thoughts for about 15 minutes; a burden was beginning to lift.

Mindful of not wanting to reinforce the negative words in those statements, I continued in a different direction with phrases such as these:

"My body is filled with joy. My body is filled with love. I nurture myself from the inside out. I accept myself as I am. I accept and love all parts of myself, and my body. I am perfect in my imperfection.

"I am safe. I am secure. I am supported (I listed several ways in which this is true). The Universe supports me. It always gives me what I need. Every experience has been, is, and will be for my benefit; there is good in every one of them."

These kinds of thoughts left me feeling a rush of appreciation for everyone who crossed my mind, including many who had hurt me. There was also a powerful sense of peace and safety, both of which I had been seeking throughout my life, not understanding that they had always been available to me. It was such a beautiful experience to realise that they're right here with me in the thoughts I choose moment to moment.

After meditating for a while on those thoughts, I continued with these:

"I move forward in my life easily, knowing that every moment is an adventure. I flow with the changes in my life, eagerly anticipating what lies around the next corner, what is in the next moment. I accept and appreciate all changes because they allow me to find out who I am and what the Universe has to offer, and what it has in store for me.

"I am flexible, changeable, flowing, moving, accepting."

I was filled with a sense of excitement and anticipation, then moved onto one of the exercises I teach in my meditation classes. I spent several minutes focusing on ideas such as these:

"I am love. I am forgiveness. I am joy. I am perfect health. I am free. I am safe. I am peace," and similar "I am..." statements.

This was, and still is, one of my favourite ways to begin — and end — the day and it has gone a long way to improving my overall health and wellbeing.

Chapter Twenty-Nine

A few more reminders of best steps toward feeling better...

Because we are 70% water, just like the Earth, remember the words of geobiologist Roy Riggs, "When you are outside, your body comes into resonance with the earth's natural voltage." Consider what Chinese medicine, other Eastern traditions and all of those tree-huggers teach about the energy that comes from the Earth. Do make an effort to get outside every day. Even if all you can do is sit on a patio or in your garden or at a nearby park, get out and reconnect with the healing energy of the Earth. Weather permitting, lie on the grass (or in the snow!) and feel the energy rushing up and into your body as you stare at the sky and watch the clouds.

Envisioning energy flowing through your body in this way is one of the key components in healing yourself. If you are not used to doing energy work, Tai Chi is an excellent way to help you get started, especially because of the physical element.

Once you've considered everything physical and external, it is time to go inward and use meditation to direct energy for purposes of healing. You may enjoy one of my guided meditation audios, such as

225

*"**Healing and Empowering Meditation**", or "**Inner Child Healing**"* (one for men, one for women), all of which are available on my website.

As I've outlined in the pages of this book, and as I've also learned in my professional background in social work and healing industries, I'm aware that there can be many reasons for our symptoms — some of which are beyond our control but it's good to know that many of them are, which is the whole point of this book. We might not always have a conscious awareness of what those reasons are, but the subconscious is sending specific messages and it's up to us to interpret them if we are going to heal whatever is wrong.

This requires reprogramming your subconscious so it will send out different messages via the neurotransmitters it creates. The first step toward achieving this is in being willing to let go of the need for the symptom, or the distressing emotion.

For example, you may be clinging to anger at someone and feel as though letting go of it is like saying you're okay with what that person did to you. It doesn't mean that at all. It just means you've chosen to stop feeling angry because it doesn't feel good and it's doing harm to your body and mind. It can be difficult to do, however, and it may be a bit of a leap to say, "I am letting go of my anger." It might be easier to say, "I am willing to let go of my anger." At least something is beginning to budge; those words allow movement and change, and can help to dislodge the emotion that is causing you pain.

It is essential, therefore, at the beginning of every meditation (even the "mini" ones) to begin by saying, "I am willing to let go of the need for _____" and name the symptom or problem. Repeat this a few times until you feel certain that the idea has settled as much as it can in that moment. Then zero in on the symptom and what it's trying to tell you, as I described having done with many of mine.

As a homeopath, I have been trained to figure out what my body was trying to tell me, and I've spent many years sorting it out for my patients. It's not always obvious but sometimes it's a lot clearer than it might seem. It might need a more objective pair of eyes to help you figure out what your body is saying.

It's a bit like learning a new language. Some words are easy to understand. Others, not so much. Think of it as a new way to see what's going on for you, how you feel about your life and the events and people that affect it. It's a bit of self-analysis, really. Begin with the part of your body that is affected and see if you can figure out how it relates to your daily life and functioning.

For example, your bones give you structure, stability. Bone problems could indicate feelings of weakness or problems in these areas. Your joints allow you to bend; they give you flexibility. Are you being rigid in areas of your life that are causing you problems? Muscles help your body move. If you have muscle pain, perhaps there is an issue with movement in your life. Are you unwilling to move forward? Are you afraid? An uncertain future can make people want to stay put whether figuratively or literally — but the truth is, the future is never certain anyway. Playing it safe by refusing to take chances or make progress in your life will not guarantee a positive result.

Breast problems can be related to issues of mother or mothering. For women who have problems with reproductive organs, menstruation etc., these can mean there are issues with femininity or the idea of sex. They can also be rooted in sexual abuse. Throat problems might be about having difficult speaking up. Maybe it's a feeling of "choking on words" and wanting to say something but not daring to do it.

Like many people, I've had some arthritis off and on in my hands, beginning when I was just 25. Hands do so many things. They touch, they hold things — and I've had massive issues and lessons about "letting go" in my life and wanting to "hold on" when it wasn't good for me. Perhaps the occasional problems with hands were the physical manifestation of this reluctance, as many people do have problems letting go of emotional issues, the past, memories and so on.

Physical pain is often a reflection of emotional pain. Once you pinpoint the grief, criticism, anger, guilt or any other unpleasant emotions to which you have been clinging, and the reasons for them, you can begin to heal.

You must also examine how your symptoms affect your life. For example, do they save you from doing things you would really rather not do? Do you have flare-ups right before events that you will find disturbing, distressing, or just plain boring? Do your symptoms keep you relying on someone else to take care of you in some way?

And if so, do you fear being independent? Are you afraid of being alone? Do you fear failure? This one can also make people ill right around exam times, or it can give them illnesses that prevent them going into jobs or professions that they would really love to pursue.

You can see it is all fairly logical, but if you are stuck, you could try browsing bookshops or looking online to find information about the meaning of specific symptoms. You could begin by looking up Chinese medicine and which emotional issues are connected to which organs.

Or check out Louise Hay's books; she is just one author who can give you some excellent ideas about healing specific ailments. She worked with people for decades, sorting out what various symptoms might mean and working out some healing affirmations that you could use in your meditations. There are others who have done similar work; you will find a lot of information about this if you begin looking for it.

Dr Phil McGraw's brilliant book "Self Matters" includes a wealth of compassionate and insightful information along with some exercises to get you digging into what makes you tick and figuring out why you do the things you do. This can also offer clues to why you have some of your particular health issues, which might help you to understand what needs healing and how to work toward healing it.

Once you've sorted out the reason(s) for your symptoms, whether you address them specifically, or your overall illness in general, repeat affirmations that begin to reprogram your subconscious and relieve it of its fears and the issues that have contributed to you being sick.

While you are repeating these statements, visualise your body being healed. In whatever ways work for you, see healing energy flowing through your body, especially settling in and around the areas that are causing you trouble. The more often you do this and the more focused you are, the better and quicker it can help.

And above all, finish every meditation with gratitude for your healing. Don't just say it; *feel* it. Thank the Universe, the God of your understanding — or even your body — whatever works for you — but feel a deep sense of gratitude for already having been healed. See yourself, in your mind's eye, doing some of those activities that are on your "to-do" list in your notebook. Gratitude is a powerfully positive emotion and has been proven time and again to help people with healing. It is not enough to just think about it or feel it momentarily now and then; it's helpful to express it. Be sure to spend a little time each day writing about your gratitude for anything, for everything, for *something*.

Do not ignore it on the bad days. Do it *especially* on the bad days. That's when you need it most — for perspective — like with that kaleidoscope. Seeing the good in your life can make the hard parts less difficult. It might sound a little corny but trust me, making sure you find aspects of your life for which to be grateful every day and writing about them even briefly can have an enormously positive impact on your ability to heal.

Chapter Thirty

Ohhhh, here's a personal favourite — a healing meditation bath. I know some people don't enjoy being in a bath at all, so let's blame my Pisces Sun for giving me a natural affinity for water. Or maybe it's simply because water is cleansing and carries with it a rich, global symbolism that can be carried into many aspects of life.

Whatever the reason, these bathing meditations are always soothing, yet powerful. Sometimes, I have one in the middle of the afternoon because I have the luxury of keeping my own hours. I light candles and sometimes turn on favourite "atmospheric" background music for a little added relaxation.

Make sure you have a bathtub cushion to support your neck so you can be as comfortable as possible. You might like to have rocks or stones in your bath, as they add a lovely grounding element, especially in terms of feng shui, and keeping your energy from "going down the drain". You could write words on the stones that reflect qualities you would like to generate or increase in yourself and your life, as I mentioned in an earlier chapter. Because of Dr Emoto's work, I find it even easier to imagine those energies flowing into and through my own body because of its water content.

Sometimes I go one step further and imagine that I am immersed, for example, in gratitude, not water. Or I tell myself that I am immersed in healing, or peace or joy. The next step is to envision that particular energy flooding through my whole body, as though I become a part of it and it is a part of me.

This is one of the most beautiful and emotional meditations I have ever done. When I've told my meditation students about it, they've often said they can't wait to get home and try it. Later, they tell me that they loved it. Some have teased about wishing they could live in the bathtub because it these meditations are so powerful and feel so wonderful.

When I began this self-healing project and was doing these bathing meditations every day, I over-filled the bathtub on purpose. Then, while keeping my feet on a large stone to ground me and connect me to Earth energy, I envisioned all negativity, self-destructive tendencies, the desire to smoke, anything harmful leaving me and rising to the surface of the water. I saw it like oily sludge and envisioned all that toxicity leaving me and rushing down the overflow drain, while everything positive remained. It was a wonderful beginning to every bath — and I have continued this practice ever since. It leaves me feeling focused, cleansed, peaceful and balanced.

Early in this project, I had quite a bad headache (as I often did back then). I thought I'd test-drive some of my new ideas and see if one of these bathing meditations would do the trick. Of course, that meant candles and soft music, and a lot of hot water. I spent ages in the tub, just kept adding more hot water, and each time I did so, I envisioned negativity, worries and the pain in my head disappearing down the overflow as I heard the water gently trickling down the drain.

Once I was out of the bath, I wrote about my gratitude for some of the many blessings in my life. Somewhere along the way, my headache had vanished. This was a far healthier option and will have had a much bigger healing effect on my entire being than just taking pain meds and getting rid of a headache.

In all things, balance is essential. We must remember the yin and yang of life; work and play, light and dark, hot and cold, seasons and cycles, everything in nature requires balance. And so it is with energy, too.

Remember, we are not human beings having a spiritual experience, we are spiritual beings having a human experience. All healing must include both the physical and the spiritual (or energetic) realms. One of my favourite meditations combines the two quite beautifully and simply. First, I envision the heavy, dense, yin energy of the Earth coming up into my feet, either through resting them on a large rock in my bath, or from the ground or the floor if I'm sitting. Second, I envision the light, expansive, yang energy from the Universe coming through my crown chakra at the top of my head.

I imagine the two meeting energies inside me, completing a circuit that connects both physical and spiritual. Together, they form sparks like millions of tiny yin/yang symbols that flow through my body while I concentrate on feeling balanced and calm.

For the duration of the meditation, I imagine a huge yin/yang symbol on each part of my body where there has been weakness or pain, for example my kidneys, while sending them messages of strength, balance and perfect healing. This technique works well for headaches, or for cold and flu symptoms such as sinus congestion and sore throat, and other complaints.

A variation on this meditation is to simply sit cross-legged with palms on knees, remembering the Tai Chi belief about "energy return", and imagine pure white healing light, or energy, flowing from above, entering your body through your crown chakra. Feel it circulate through your body, and see if you notice it settling in any particular part or parts. When I began doing this at the beginning of this project, I felt it settling and swirling in my hips and pelvis, just like after the first time I did the P.M. Tai Chi workout.

To be honest, I'm still amazed by how quickly and dramatically I noticed improvement in that part of my body. The terrible, gnawing pain that used to wake me several times every night had vanished and I was able to walk — and fairly briskly, too — without anything more than the occasional slight grumble from my hip.

If you're feeling stuck and don't know where to begin, below are some ideas for you to consider while meditating. Pick whichever one(s) fit or change them to suit your needs:

I am MEANT TO BE HERE - JUST LIKE EVERYONE ELSE on the planet. My existence is a joyous and beautiful thing.

I am a survivor. I will always survive. I am okay. I have always been okay.

I am precious. I am special. I am valuable. I am important. I matter. I love every part of myself, inside and out, my good points and my not so good points because they are all part of me. I am a work in progress, and I am lovable. I am perfect.

I am valuable. I am important. I matter.

I accept and I love all parts of myself.

I am safe. I am loved. I am safe. I am loved. I am safe. I am loved...

My mistakes do not define me. I am an imperfect human and I am always doing my best. Therefore, I can release all guilt for things that have gone wrong, for choices that turned out badly, for times when I did not have the wisdom to handle things better. I can release the guilt, and along with it, the need for the pain it causes.

*I am grateful to be able to experience life and its beauty. I am grateful for the many blessings in my life (spend some time thinking about them and **feeling** the gratitude).*

Or you might try one of my favourites, a very simple little morning meditation that I do sometimes before getting out of bed. This one's super simple.

Sit up in bed and hug yourself. Wrap your arms around your upper body, gently stroking your back, sides, arms, with genuine affection as you tell your body "I love you." Say it like you mean it, as though you were talking to a child you love dearly.

Draw your knees up to your chest if you are able, put your arms around them and include your legs in the hug. Feel a flood of love and joy flow through you. Connect with a deep appreciation for your body and all it does for you. Allow yourself to feel peaceful, safe and secure. If you've never known these, how beautiful it will be to discover that they are right there in your hands.

It will be essential for you to spend some time every day purely meditating on the belief that you are well, that you are healed, cured, or fully recovered. At first, you might feel like a liar saying such things. Your fear of never recovering might pipe up and try to sabotage your efforts by telling you something quite different.

Chase it away by reminding yourself of Morris Goodman, or the Qigong medicine-less hospital wiping out a 3-inch tumour in a matter of minutes. Think about all those people with Dissociative Identity Disorder, whose bodies respond immediately to the belief that there are tumours, burns, scars, epilepsy — whatever — and can either create or eliminate them.

It might take some time for you to get used to new and positive thoughts, but the more often you choose them, the easier it becomes. You will be well on your way to reprogramming your subconscious by changing your belief system, which is an essential key to improving your health.

The amount of time you spend in focused meditations is entirely up to you but obviously, the more you do it, the better it will work. You might want to start with 5-10 minutes at a time, but I would suggest that you should aim for a minimum of 20-30 minutes, once or twice a day. Any time in between that you can manage even a brief period of positive, healing imagery or self-talk will help. You can do it while sitting at a red light, waiting in a queue, doing the washing up after a meal or even while brushing your teeth. Your health matters enough to you that you are reading this book. I assume, then, that it matters enough that you're willing to make some lifestyle changes and create new habits.

In theory, self-healing *can* be simple but it won't happen overnight. The more effort you put into it, the better your results will be. It takes discipline to make positive changes consistently so they become a regular part of your day and contribute to your wellbeing. Doesn't that sound delicious? Of course it does. A common stumbling block for many is "I'm too busy." Too busy for even a short walk? Too busy for 10-15 minutes of Tai Chi, yoga, or quiet meditation?

Too busy to choose better thoughts? That one doesn't even require extra time.

And they wonder why they have become ill.

Your body doesn't care about deadlines or housework or other obligations, some of which are likely to be self-inflicted. The truth is, this is about priorities and understanding that if you don't put your health first, everything else will fall apart at some point.

In many cases, it isn't so much that people are "too busy". It's that they are too tired or would rather watch their favourite shows on the telly, or scroll on their phones. How many times have you heard people say that time just vanishes when they're playing on the internet or social media? A couple of hours go by in a blink.

Are those activities worth more than your health?

As for having too much to do, learn to delegate where possible. Ask for help. Accept the fact that dust bunnies under the bed will wait for you and no earthly harm will come to you because of them. If you really want to be well, then you have to make it your number one priority and get on with it.

The bottom line is that if you're not okay, there will come a point where other aspects of your life won't be okay either.

We will always make time for whatever is important in our lives. It is not hard to carve out at 30-60 minutes out of every 24 hours to go inward, heal, restore and rejuvenate yourself — mind, body and soul. In fact, incorporating many of the suggestions in this book, such as improving nutrition and activity levels, and perhaps taking a short power-nap here and there, don't even have to take a lot of time but they can increase your energy levels — and therefore, your productivity — fairly quickly.

I had been working at this self-healing project for about eight months when I had occasion to be hooked up to a complicated bit of technology that would evaluate my cardiovascular and autonomic nervous systems. It measured several aspects of each one, and even included an ECG and detail about what the results meant.

As I'd been working on my self-healing project, I was delighted to have an opportunity to test it with some objectivity. I had been feeling increasingly well and was no longer having any problems that impeded my ability to live a normal life. I didn't hurt; my joint and muscle pain was gone. It was impossible to walk any faster without preparing for take-off. I knew I was vastly improved on all levels. But still, I was excited by the idea of obtaining test results that could not be disputed.

For months, I had been meditating and visualising and focusing on my heart being healed, and functioning beautifully. Although I had been feeling so much better overall, I was fully prepared to see a fair bit of residual heart attack damage, given that it had shown up on thallium scans several years earlier. After all, I had been pretty sick for such a long time and although my symptoms had disappeared, I had only been doing this self-healing work for a few months and wasn't expecting miracles.

How shocked was I to discover that most of the results for cardio-vascular function were within normal range, and a couple of them were even "optimal". The test was run twice that evening, and two aspects of the ECG were minimally diminished the second time, but still within "normal" range. Blood circulation and artery health were at Level 2 ("good", with Level 1 being "great", and Level 7 being "why are you still breathing?"). My blood pressure, which had been at the borderline worrisome place for some time, was a very healthy 105/68.

And...I could not believe my eyes when I looked at my pulse rate. For much of my life, my heart would pound and race like mad on a regular basis. My pulse was more often in the high 80s or low 90s than anywhere else. The first column on the graph showed age ranges, and beside it were seven more columns showing pulse rate ranges for each: Athletes, Excellent, Good, Above Average and so on down to Poor. I hoped I could at least make it to the mid-way point with Average.

My pulse, ranging between 57 and 60, was in the column marked "Athletes".

Clearly, my self-healing project was working. To be honest, I had not expected such dramatic improvements, at least not so soon. I was encouraged to continue with everything I'd been doing, and especially meditating to visualise healing and energy work, which was the most powerful piece of the entire puzzle. My health had improved vastly on all levels. The disturbing and violent nightmares had stopped, and although I would always miss England terribly, I was no longer being eaten alive by homesickness or the painfully sad dreams I'd been experiencing.

On top of that, meditation is its own reward, even without the added health benefits it can bring. I've heard this from many people over the years, including my students, who sometimes squawk in the early days about having a hard time setting aside even 5-10 minutes of meditation every day. But once they get the hang of meditating and experience the joy and peace they find in those minutes, they want more. It's like flossing your teeth or taking up any other habit that is new; it just takes a bit of time to make it a regular part of your day. Once you get to that point, if you miss your usual meditation, you will feel it right away.

You aren't doing any of this for anyone else. You are doing it for yourself. The more you put into this self-healing project, the more you will get out of it. Do you really want to feel better? Your body is screaming at you for a break, for a large dose of positive input, and some tender loving care. It is reflecting the physical, mental and emotional environments to which it has been subjected for a long time and it's pleading with you for help.

I don't want you to beat yourself up about this. All of us do the best we can with whatever circumstances and information we have at any given time. It doesn't help that most of us realise, at least in part, that we're not always taking care of ourselves as well as we could, but we carry on anyway with the less-than-wonderful diet, the ingestion of toxic substances, a lack of exercise.

We continue to surround ourselves with negative people, we stew in our stifled resentments, we choke back our tears. All too often, we stay up later than we should, and on top of these other self-destructive behaviours, we wonder why we're so exhausted from one day to the next. We know we could do things a little better, but to a large extent, we think we are immortal, or that we will worry about it later. We don't understand just how much damage we're doing to our health because of some of the choices we make.

Please allow yourself to accept that you've done the best you could with the information you had, but now you have new information that will allow you to make healthier choices in every aspect of your life, beginning with the thoughts you feed your subconscious. Reprogramming the belief systems that have been planted in it, and that have a significant impact on your health and life, is easiest when you are in a deep state of relaxation, reducing distractions and focusing on what you want to achieve.

If your illness has taken over your life, if you feel like you've *become* your illness, you can begin by recognising that it is *not* part of your identity. You are a person who has become ill, and must see yourself this way as a first step in taking control of your life and your health again. It is essential to begin taking steps to get your thoughts out of the hole that you've found yourself in, the one that is just a big cesspool of illness with you stuck down the bottom of it.

If your life revolves mainly — or largely — around your illness and how it's adversely affecting you, one way you can help to shift away from that focus is to see if you can help others who need assistance in some way. Or just take an active interest in the lives of those around you. Allow some of the outside world back into your life. Your own world may have become quite small if you have been ill and restricted for some time. Try to find ways to open a window or a door again, let some light in — and let yourself out. It's a great way to gain some perspective about your own issues.

At the very least, take up a hobby. Pick up a long-forgotten one. Get interested in something that isn't about your illness. Find something to do that occupies your brain, your energy, and your thoughts in a positive way. Find ways to be creative, and don't worry about what anyone else thinks about the results. One of the points of it is to express yourself and release whatever has been buried inside you for some time, perhaps always. An even bigger point is just to have some fun. Yeah, fun. Remember what that is?

We hear people talk about that "little voice" inside, that nagging "something" in our guts that will often poke its head up and give us messages that more often than not, many of us ignore. Later, we discover that we've made a mistake; the little voice had been right and we should have listened to it. But time and time again, we don't. We've been taught not to trust that little voice, or to ignore it because we do not trust ourselves. Or that other people's needs are more important than our own. We succumb to peer pressure or to the opinions of others, perhaps because we want their approval or we are avoiding confrontation, or for one of a million other reasons.

That little voice that speaks to you is your highest self. It is your spirit and knows what is right and best for you. It tries to speak above the noise of Ego, which is your human self, the part of you that gets caught up in hurt feelings, or worries about others' expectations of you. Ego-generated thoughts also make you feel guilty, ashamed, angry, jealous, resentful and fearful. These are the kinds thoughts that create toxic energy, and toxic chemical messages that make you ill.

Learning to listen to the tiny voice of your highest self is one of the most healing, beneficial and empowering things you can do for yourself.

Recently, a friend was trying to make a difficult decision. To be more specific, she had made the decision but was wrestling with whether or not she dared follow through. I told her to listen to that little voice and it would never lie. The next time we spoke, she said the little voice she heard was all about shoulds and shouldn'ts and what her various family members wanted from her.

I told her that that's *not* the voice of her highest self. That's simply ego — her human side — the mother, daughter, and wife that was listening to other people's expectations, needs and demands of her.

Your highest self — that little voice inside — it will tell you how you really feel and what you want. It's about *what's best for you*, not anyone else.

The best way to hear your truth is to ask yourself, "What do I really need? How do I really feel? What do I really want?"

Then remove everyone else from the equation as you listen for the answers. If they are about what someone else wants from you, that's not the little voice that will never steer you wrong. Push aside other people's needs and let your own truth come shining through. Then, and only then, should you make a decision.

In the end, the more you take care of yourself, the better off you will be on all levels. Ultimately, this will allow you to be more and do more for all of those people who rely on you and want you to be a part of their lives.

Trust yourself. Respect yourself. Honour yourself. Your body— and everyone you love — will thank you for it.

Chapter Thirty-One

There have been so many powerful experiences and pieces of information that have gone into the creation of this book. It is impossible to pick out any one of them as being at the top of the list when considering whether or not self-healing is possible for everyone, and not just a rare and lucky few. But if I had to choose just one, it might be in one simple, yet powerful fact about our very existence.

We know that all living organisms are hard-wired for survival. It is tied up in DNA, cell intelligence, the instincts of even the tiniest insect that just "knows" what to do, how to live, how to reproduce. The "default setting" of any organism is to be healthy; it is not a natural state to be ill. Therefore, whether a fruit fly, a rose bush, or a human being, in order to survive, there must be an inherent ability for the organism to withstand numerous attacks from outside sources of all kinds, from the teeth and claws of vicious predators, to bacteria, and so much more.

Every day, we must deal with the fallout of modern life and its stresses, its environmental toxins and pollutants, our growing list of genetically modified foods. There are plenty of attacks on our bodies,

dreams and happiness — or they'll help strengthen the destructive beliefs that derail you.

Ultimately, changing your thoughts will change your life — if that is what you choose.

It is true that we create our own realities. If we see ourselves as worthless and believe that we will never amount to anything, that's going to have a direct impact on the results we get. If we believe life is filled with good things and happiness, then we'll naturally steer ourselves down paths that will give us what we envisioned and we'll notice all the good along the way.

Speaking of being steered down a path... Somewhere in the midst of working on this book, while I was out for my walk one morning, my thoughts drifted back to a deeply private and profound experience I'd had several years earlier. After it happened, I knew how it would sound if I actually told anyone about it, and given my mental state at the time I was afraid of the possible repercussions. So I kept it to myself and never told a soul for years. Even then, I only shared it with only a handful of people closest to me. But now I must share it with you.

It was a misty, grey, February morning in England a long time ago - several years before the events that led to this self-healing project. I was in the midst of something of an emotional meltdown after an overload of crises and stress. My father had died just a few weeks earlier, and there were frightening and difficult family issues happening at the same time. It was all a bit much, and unusually, I cracked under the strain. It wasn't like me to come apart, even in the face of a lot of emotional pressure.

I went for a walk around the lake that was just a stone's throw from Ravenswood. Deep in thought, I was unaware of my surroundings as I stared at the ground, putting one foot in front of the other. That was pretty much how I had lived most of my life, really — just getting through what was immediately in front of me, unable to cope with looking at anything else as I made my way through one crisis after another.

With my hands shoved into my pockets and my head hanging, everything about me drooped at least as much as my spirit. Sighing heavily, I trudged along, the weight of the world on my shoulders. My heart was so heavy; I felt so lost. Damaged. Utterly broken.

Halfway around the lake, I found a fallen tree nestled into the woods, just at the water's edge. Stepping over rocks and branches, I wept silently as I made my way to the log and sat down. I thought I might weep forever as overwhelming sadness and pain bubbled up from the very depths of my soul, spilling forth and unstoppable.

"Please, please, *please* heal me!" I whispered, tears streaming down my face as I wrapped my arms tightly around myself and rocked back and forth ever so gently. Just who I thought might be listening to my desperate plea was anyone's guess but on the chance that there was a Divine Being out there who might actually exist and hear me, I had to try.

"I've had such a lot of stress and pain in my life," I whispered. "I can't take this any more. I am so ill, so broken, in such despair! Please, please will you heal me? Please please please! Please will you take away this pain and make me whole?"

As I sat on that log, hugging myself and rocking back and forth, the same thoughts kept spinning round and round in my head. 'I am so horribly, desperately alone and ill ill ill right to my core, to the centre of my very soul, I will never be well, never be healed, never move beyond this misery!'

And then the most incredible thing happened.

There I was, pleading with "the Universe" — or some nameless, non-specific Source of Creation that may or may not exist — to heal me, to take away my pain, when suddenly, I swear I felt a powerful Presence immediately above me. It descended and surrounded me completely.

In an instant, I began to vibrate as though a thousand volts raced through my body, entering at the top of my head and running right the way down my body, through my feet and into the ground and back up again like lightning, tearing up and down, up and down, causing me to tremble visibly.

It was a much tamer version of the sensation I experienced when I was healing someone, only far more powerful than I had ever experienced before. I was frightened, bewildered — to be honest, I was freaking out because if I believed what I thought was happening, then maybe I really *had* snapped.

And then I heard words. I heard them deep inside myself. "Yes. Yes, you will be healed. You are a healer. You have great work to do. You are meant to heal many people."

First, I was shocked to get an answer.

Second, I was puzzled about what it meant.

I had a vague thought about it possibly meaning a return to practicing homeopathy. Without actually posing the question, an answer came. "No. You are meant to heal on a much wider scale than that. You will find the path that allows you to heal masses of people."

I knew that sounded nuts and I knew it sounded arrogant. And I knew I was neither. At least, I was pretty sure I wasn't nuts, although to be honest, in the midst of that entire experience I was questioning it.

Then a thought: What if that answer was the truth?

Nah. Couldn't be. "But how?" I whispered. It didn't help that I felt completely broken and lost. I couldn't seem to pull myself together; how on earth would I ever heal "masses of people"?

And then came the qualifier. "But first, you must heal yourself."

Um... yeah. No kidding. I mean, I was hanging on by a thread; there was no way I could help anyone else at that point. I wondered if that meant I needed to get back to regular meditation, spiritual practice, some yoga, that sort of thing, as they'd fallen by the wayside with the circumstances in my life and family situations. Maybe it meant I was supposed to give myself a big rest after a load of stress and soon I'd be good to go again.

Something inside me knew it meant much more than that. But what on earth could I ever do that would help "masses of people"?

Still in the midst of the power surge and feeling that Presence, I was struggling to absorb the experience.

'I can't tell anyone about this!' I thought. 'I'll sound crazy! I'll be locked up! But I *know* this is happening. This is *not* my imagination.'

Yet I realised that if I *had* been crazy, I wouldn't have known it. I wouldn't have been afraid to tell anyone about this incredible experience. I was still vibrating with that frighteningly powerful surge of energy running up and down through my body and I knew I couldn't make *that* up.

'Boy, you really are having a meltdown, aren't you?' I thought, nervously laughing at myself but fearing this had been Step One in slipping off my pulley. 'Well, calm down. You can chalk this up to having some sort of weird religious experience out of your dark and terrible desperation, and you don't have to worry about being a few bricks short of a load. But you know you're going to believe this was the real deal, don't you? Because it is.'

It was several minutes before the tears slowed, the vibrating stopped, and the Presence left me. Stunned and overwhelmed by the whole experience, it was a long time before I could leave that hidden place by the water and return to Ravenswood, knowing I would never be the same.

Fast forward several years... I was out walking one morning during this project and writing this book. It had been years since I'd thought about that day at the lake. Suddenly, there it was in my head, an image of myself sitting on that log, desperate beyond words. I remembered my tearful, tormented plea to be healed and the answer that had come back, telling me yes, I would be healed, because I was meant to heal many others.

I thought about the twists and turns of my life since then, a course that had most definitely not allowed me to heal anywhere near "masses of people".

As I walked, I remembered the most crucial words of all: *First, I had to heal myself.*

I nearly stopped in my tracks. Finally, I understood.

I'd been told that I would find the path that would allow me to heal many other people. In that moment, I realised that this was it. My self-healing project, everything that eventually led me to write this book, this is at least a part of what was meant that day at the lake so long ago.

That path did not begin with my frustrated outburst and vow to heal myself after I moved back to Calgary. Nor did it begin with my decision to write this book. It didn't even begin that day at the lake.

It began a lifetime ago and has been creating itself with every experience, every ailment, every bit of suffering, every heartbreak, every medical appointment or treatment I've had. The path has included countless bits of reading and study, personal and professional experience, conversations, investigations and a whole load of curiosity and research over many years. There have been so many random pieces of information that I learned along that path, combined with countless new ones while working on figuring out how to heal myself and sharing them in this book.

All of them have come together to create this one magnificent picture of hope so I could share it with you and help you on your road to healing and wellness.

I want to leave you with one delicious little suggestion that you might want to use daily. It is the Buddhist "Smiling Meditation". There are many ways you can do it; a bit of research will yield several results, I'm sure. But the short version is that you will just quietly with your eyes closed and smile. Notice how the smile feels. Think about how it spreads. Your cheeks are smiling. Your chin is smiling. Your ears are smiling. Your eyes, your eyebrows, even your hair is smiling.

Work your way down as the smile spreads all through your body, externally as well as internally. Imagine your lungs smiling, your ribs, your elbows, spleen, liver, kidneys. Imagine your heart has a big smile plastered right in the center of it. Even your knees are smiling.

Every cell in your body is smiling. Your blood cells are smiling. I like to think of them as little happy faces zipping through my body.

Do this as often and as long as the mood hits. You can do this one briefly any time you think about it — while you're "on hold" on the phone or waiting in a queue or sitting at the dentist's office (an extra good place to relax!). Take a few seconds or maybe a few minutes and simply focus on every part of your body smiling.

The interesting thing about this meditation is that even if you are feeling anything but smiley when you begin, the very act of putting a smile on your face and holding it for a short time will actually cause your brain to get the message that you are smiling. In turn, it releases wonderfully calming and mood-elevating chemical messengers that are sent throughout your body. Soon, you will actually feel lighter and happier than before you started.

Finish with gratitude, as with your other meditations. Take a few moments and feel how wonderful it is to be happy, to be smiling. Consider the many blessings in your life. This, in and of itself, is deeply healing all by itself.

There's so much more that could have been included within these pages. I didn't want to overwhelm you. At least you have been given a powerful and empowering starting point, a place to begin your own investigations. You can test-drive my suggestions and alter them so they work for you.

There is a wealth of information out there, more help, more detail, more evidence, more suggestions — whatever you need to support your journey to wellness. But the most important source of all — the most powerful source of your healing — is right there, safely tucked away inside you, just waiting for you to discover it and create your very own miracle.

Bon voyage!

Bibliography

REFERENCES FOR "THE POWER AND SIMPLICITY OF SELF-HEALING":

Below is a partial list of the various resources that were used in the writing of this book. Much of the information came from accumulated learning throughout my life in terms of my training and experience. Some of it came from a lot of research on the internet.

When I set out on this journey, I had no idea that I would achieve the results I did or that my experience would become a book. Therefore, I didn't keep track of the many sources of information I found.

Apologies for only being able to provide a partial list.

The Miracle of Water, by Masaru Emoto

The Hidden Messages in Water, by Masaru Emoto

Quantum Healing, by Deepak Chopra

The Forces Behind Feng Shui, by Dawn Hankins

The Western Guide to Feng Shui: Room by Room, by Terah Kathryn Collins

What Your Doctor Doesn't Know About Nutritional Medicine May Be Killing You, by Ray Strand MD

The Power of Your Subconscious Mind, by Dr Joseph Murray

Between Heaven and Earth - A Guide To Chinese Medicine, Harriet Beinfield and Efrem Korngold

When Rabbit Howls, by Truddi Chase

Life Extension Magazine, Julius G Goepp MD, May 2008

Discover Magazine, August 2000, Dr T Colin Campbell, PhD

Arizona Center for Advanced Medicine, an article by Dr Samuel S Epstein, author of *What's In Your Milk*

The Physicians Committee for Responsible Medicine, Neal Barnard, head of PCRM

"Nitric Oxide is 'molecule of the year'" 19 December 1992, article by Steve Connor in The Independent

The Legacy of Alfred Nobel, R. Sohlman, The Bodley Head Ltd. London 1983

Buijsse B., Feskens EJM, Kok FJ, Kromhout D, *Cocoa intake, blood pressure and cardiovascular mortality: the Zutphen Elderly Study*. Arch Intern Med 2006; 166:411-7.

Wyatt DA, Ely SW, Lasley RD, et al. *Purine-enriched asanguineous cardioplegia retards adenosine triphosphate degradation during ischemia and improves postischemic ventricular function*. J Thorac Cardiovascular Surgeon 1989 May; 97(5):771-8.

Wolverton Environmental Services, Inc. wolvertonenvironmental.com

249

Bibliography

World Health Organisation website: www.who.int

Harvard health blog, www.health.harvard.edu/blog/mindfulness-meditation-improves-connections-in-the-brain-201104082253

www.abc-of-yoga.com/meditation/benefits.asp

www.dailymail.co.uk

www.telegraph.co.uk

www.royriggs.co.uk

www.bodyecology.com

Nobelprize.org - official website of the Nobel Prize

www.webmd.com

Numerous other websites

About the Author

Liberty Forrest is an award-winning author of several books. Her non-fiction books are on self-help topics and even include an inspirational colouring book.

She has also written several later-in-life, small-town clean romance novels under the pen name, Ruby Ashford.

Currently, Liberty enjoys a quiet life in Western Canada.

Follow Liberty on Patreon (it's free).

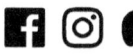